Treating the Adult Neurogenic Bladder

Guest Editors

JOHN T. STOFFEL, MD
EDWARD J. MCGUIRE, MD

UROLOGIC CLINICS OF NORTH AMERICA

www.urologic.theclinics.com

November 2010 • Volume 37 • Number 4

SAUNDERS an imprint of ELSEVIER, Inc.

W.B. SAUNDERS COMPANY
A Division of Elsevier Inc.

1600 John F. Kennedy Blvd. • Suite 1800 • Philadelphia, PA 19103-2899

http://www.theclinics.com

UROLOGIC CLINICS OF NORTH AMERICA Volume 37, Number 4
November 2010 ISSN 0094-0143, ISBN-13: 978-1-4377-2535-3

Editor: Kerry Holland
Developmental Editor: Jessica Demetriou

Urologic Clinics of North America (ISSN 0094-0143) is published quarterly by Elsevier Inc., 360 Park Avenue South, New York, NY 10010-1710. Months of issue are February, May, August, and November. Business and Editorial Offices: 1600 John F. Kennedy Blvd., Suite 1800, Philadelphia, PA 19103-2899. Periodicals postage paid at New York, NY and additional mailing offices. Subscription prices are $311.00 per year (US individuals), $519.00 per year (US institutions), $363.00 per year (Canadian individuals), $636.00 per year (Canadian institutions), $451.00 per year (foreign individuals), and $636.00 per year (foreign institutions). Foreign air speed delivery is included in all *Clinics* subscription prices. All prices are subject to change without notice. **POSTMASTER:** Send address changes to *Urologic Clinics of North America*, Elsevier Health Sciences Division, Subscription Customer Service, 3251 Riverport Lane, Maryland Heights, MO 63043. Customer Service: 1-800-654-2452 (US). From outside the United States, call 1-314-447-8871. Fax: 1-314-447-8029. E-mail: JournalsCustomerServiceusa@elsevier.com (for print support) and JournalsOnlineSupport-usa@elsevier.com (for online support).

Reprints. For copies of 100 or more, of articles in this publication, please contact the Commercial Reprints Department, Elsevier Inc., 360 Park Avenue South, New York, New York 10010-1710. Tel.: 212-633-3813; Fax: 212-462-1935; E-mail: reprints@elsevier.com.

Urologic Clinics of North America is covered in MEDLINE/PubMed (*Index Medicus*), *Excerpta Medica, Current Contents/Clinical Medicine, Science Citation Index,* and *ISI/BIOMED*.

Printed and bound in the United Kingdom
Transferred to Digital Print 2011

Contributors

GUEST EDITORS

JOHN T. STOFFEL, MD
Associate Professor, Tufts University School of Medicine; Vice Chairman, Department of Urology, Lahey Clinic, Burlington, Massachusetts

EDWARD J. MCGUIRE, MD
Professor of Surgery, Department of Urology, University of Michigan School of Medicine, Ann Arbor, Michigan

AUTHORS

DON T. BUI, MD
Resident, Department of Urology, William Beaumont Hospital, Royal Oak, Michigan

FRANK N. BURKS, MD
Resident, Department of Urology, William Beaumont Hospital, Royal Oak, Michigan

ANNE P. CAMERON, MD, FRCPS(C)
Assistant Professor, Department of Urology, University of Michigan, Ann Arbor, Michigan

SUNG YONG CHO, MD
Department of Urology, Seoul National University College of Medicine, Seoul National University Hospital, Seoul, Korea

J. QUENTIN CLEMENS, MD, FACS, MSCI
Associate Professor of Urology, Director, Division of Neurourology and Pelvic Reconstructive Surgery, Department of Urology, University of Michigan Medical Center, Ann Arbor, Michigan

CATHERINE DALTON, MRCPI
Senior Clinical Research Associate, Department of Neuroinflammation, UCL Institute of Neurology, London, United Kingdom

CLARE J. FOWLER, FRCP
Professor of Uro-Neurology, UCL Institute of Neurology; Consultant, National Hospital for Neurology and Neurosurgery, University College London Hospital, London, United Kingdom

E. ANN GORMLEY, MD
Professor of Surgery (Urology); Program Director Urology Residency, Section of Urology, Department of Surgery, Dartmouth-Hitchcock Medical Center, Lebanon, New Hampshire

SEONG JIN JEONG, MD
Associate Professor, Department of Urology, Seoul National University Bundang Hospital, Gyeonggi-do, Korea

WENDY W. LENG, MD
Associate Professor, Department of Urology, University of Pittsburgh School of Medicine, Pittsburgh, Pennsylvania

EDWARD J. MCGUIRE, MD
Professor of Surgery, Department of Urology, University of Michigan School of Medicine, Ann Arbor, Michigan

MAJID MIRZAZADEH, MD
Instructor, Department of Urology, Wake Forest University School of Medicine, Winston-Salem, North Carolina

ARTHUR MOURTZINOS, MD
Department of Urology, Lahey Clinic, Tufts University School of Medicine, Burlington, Massachusetts

SEUNG-JUNE OH, MD
Professor, Department of Urology, Seoul National University College of Medicine, Seoul National University Hospital, Seoul, Korea

JALESH N. PANICKER, MD, DM, MRCP (UK)
Consultant Neurologist, Department of Uro-Neurology, National Hospital for Neurology and Neurosurgery, UCL Institute of Neurology, London, United Kingdom

KENNETH M. PETERS, MD
Chairman, Department of Urology, William Beaumont Hospital, Royal Oak, Michigan

BENJAMIN T. RISTAU, MD
Department of Urology, University of Pittsburgh School of Medicine, Pittsburgh, Pennsylvania

MARC C. SMALDONE, MD
Department of Urology, University of Pittsburgh School of Medicine, Pittsburgh, Pennsylvania

JOHN J. SMITH III, MD
Professor and Director Clinical Research, Department of Urology, Wake Forest University School of Medicine, Winston-Salem, North Carolina

IRINA STANASEL, MD
PGY-3, Department of Urology, Wake Forest University School of Medicine, Winston-Salem, North Carolina

JOHN T. STOFFEL, MD
Associate Professor, Tufts University School of Medicine; Vice Chairman, Department of Urology, Lahey Clinic, Burlington, Massachusetts

O. LENAINE WESTNEY, MD
Associate Professor and Fellowship Director, Urinary Tract and Pelvic Reconstruction, Department of Urology, MD Anderson Cancer Center, Houston, Texas

Contents

Preface xi

John T. Stoffel and Edward J. McGuire

Basic Bladder Neurophysiology 487

J. Quentin Clemens

Maintenance of normal lower urinary tract function is a complex process that requires coordination between the central nervous system and the autonomic and somatic components of the peripheral nervous system. This article provides an overview of the basic principles that are recognized to regulate normal urine storage and micturition, including bladder biomechanics, relevant neuroanatomy, neural control of lower urinary tract function, and the pharmacologic processes that translate the neural signals into functional results. Finally, the emerging role of the urothelium as a sensory structure is discussed.

Pharmacologic Therapy for the Neurogenic Bladder 495

Anne P. Cameron

This article is a review of the current and past literature on medical management of the neurogenic bladder, with a particular focus on spinal cord injury and multiple sclerosis. The use of antimuscarinics, α-blocker, and tricyclic antidepressants and their combined use are discussed along with new therapies in human and animal trials.

Urodynamics of the Neurogenic Bladder 507

Edward J. McGuire

Many patients with neurogenic bladders require careful monitoring in order to decrease the risk of infectious and renal complications. Urodynamic testing, with particular attention paid to detrusor pressures, is helpful for risk stratification in these patients and provides key information when assessing effectiveness of treatments. This article reviews the history, indications, and contemporary parameters for urodynamic testing in the neurogenic population.

Review of Neurologic Diseases for the Urologist 517

Clare J. Fowler, Catherine Dalton, and Jalesh N. Panicker

This article reviews the neurologic conditions associated with a high prevalence of bladder dysfunction and about which significant advances in understanding have occurred in recent years. The importance of the frontal lobes for bladder control has been confirmed through functional brain imaging, and recent findings in the elderly with incontinence suggest the problem may result from disconnection of important frontal areas caused by white matter disease. The very different urologic profile of the two sometimes-confused conditions, multiple system atrophy and Parkinson's disease, is clarified. The advances in treatments for multiple sclerosis in recent years have been remarkable and are briefly described.

Management Goals for the Spina Bifida Neurogenic Bladder: A Review from Infancy to Adulthood 527

Arthur Mourtzinos and John T. Stoffel

Patients with spina bifida require longitudinal urological care as they transition from childhood to adolescence and then to adulthood. Issues important to urological health, such as protection of the upper tracts and prevention of incontinence, need vigilant follow-up throughout the patient's life. As the child ages, additional issues such as sexual functioning also become increasingly important for social integration. Despite this need for regular assessment, many adult patients with spina bifida lose coordinated urological care after leaving specialized pediatric spina bifida clinics. Consequently, urologists frequently encounter an adult patient with spina bifida in practice and they need to understand the basic urological treatment goals and potential complications for this population.

Spinal Cord/Brain Injury and the Neurogenic Bladder **537**

Seong Jin Jeong, Sung Yong Cho, and Seung-June Oh

This article reviews neurogenic bladder related to traumatic injury as well as vascular lesion of brain/spinal cord. Because urological manifestations of traumatic or vascular brain/spinal cord injury are highly diversified and complex, the approaches to achieve accurate diagnosis and administer proper treatment can be complicated. The goal of primary treatment is preservation of renal function and attainment of social continence. Maintaining low intravesical pressure and adequate bladder emptying are central to the treatment strategy. Diagnosis and appropriate urological management of these disease entities should depend on urodynamic studies because of poor correlation between clinical symptoms or somatic neurologic signs and urodynamic findings.

Contemporary Management of the Neurogenic Bladder for Multiple Sclerosis Patients **547**

John T. Stoffel

Urinary symptoms related to multiple sclerosis (MS) present a complex challenge for the treating physician. However, several treatment options are available for the symptomatic patient once the physician understands basic MS disease epidemiology and pathophysiology. Depending of disease status and symptoms, MS urinary symptoms may respond to directed behavioral, pharmacologic, intravesical, neuromodulation, or surgical therapies.

Neuromodulation and the Neurogenic Bladder **559**

Frank N. Burks, Don T. Bui, and Kenneth M. Peters

Neurogenic bladder resulting from spinal cord injury and spina bifida has a profound impact on voiding function. This article reviews the current literature with regards to electrical stimulation for neurogenic bladder and the clinical outcomes associated with sacral neuromodulation, pudendal neuromodulation, posterior tibial nerve stimulation, and the Finetech-Brindley posterior/anterior stimulator. In addition, the world literature reviewing hemilaminectomy and ventral root micro anastomosis is discussed. The article also examines the safety of magnetic resonance imaging in patients with implanted neurostimulators and discusses common complications. Neuromodulation, both electrical and physical, play an important role in the management of neurogenic bladder.

Botulinum Toxin Therapy for Neurogenic Detrusor Overactivity **567**

Marc C. Smaldone, Benjamin T. Ristau, and Wendy W. Leng

Detrusor injection of botulinum toxin (BTX) has shown great promise in the treatment of neurogenic detrusor overactivity (NDO) refractory to conservative therapy. Despite a paucity of prospective evidence, there exists a growing consensus that BTX injection therapy is a well-tolerated, low-risk therapy. Injections result in substantial subjective improvement in continence and quality of life. Moreover, assessment of urodynamic parameters demonstrates objective changes: (1) an increase in maximum cystometric capacity; (2) when applicable, a reduction in maximal detrusor voiding pressures; and (3) an increase in bladder compliance in cases where baseline bladder compliance measures were abnormal. While BTX bladder injection offers both objective and subjective measures of incontinence control, treatment duration is limited by the gradual reinnervation of injected tissue over an approximately 6- to 9-month interval. However, repeat injection cycles do appear to achieve similar levels of efficacy. The objective of this review is to provide a focused summary of the current body of literature, investigating the safety and efficacy of bladder BTX injection in patients with NDO.

The Neurogenic Bladder and Incontinent Urinary Diversion **581**

O. Lenaine Westney

Management of the neurogenic bladder with an incontinent stoma is necessary in situations in which intermittent catheterization via the urethra or a continent stoma is not feasible. Cutaneous ureterostomy, vesicostomy, ileal conduit, and ileovesicostomy have all been used for this purpose. Vesicostomy is most commonly used as a temporizing measure in the pediatric neurogenic population. Both ileal conduit, with or without cystectomy, and ileovesicostomy have contemporary roles in the management of the neurogenic bladder.

Bladder Tissue Engineering **593**

Irina Stanasel, Majid Mirzazadeh, and John J. Smith III

The bladder can lose the ability to store and empty effectively as a result of numerous conditions. When conservative methods to maximize patient safety and quality of life fail, surgical reconstruction of the bladder is usually considered. Augmentation cystoplasty can be performed with the use of the small bowel, large bowel, or less often, stomach. An alternative approach, tissue engineering, identifies the body's own potential for regeneration and supports this propensity with appropriate raw materials and growth factors so that the body's original structure and function may be restored. Tissue engineering can involve the use of a scaffold or matrix alone or of cell-seeded matrices. Harvesting cells and culturing them has become an important tool in tissue engineering. Multiple possibilities for sources of cells have been investigated, including stem cells and differentiated cells from organs other than the bladder; however, to date, autologous bladder cells remain the gold standard for culture and seeding.

Urologic Complications of the Neurogenic Bladder **601**

E. Ann Gormley

Patients with a neurogenic bladder are at risk for several urologic complications including hydronephrosis, vesicoureteral reflux, renal failure, urinary tract infections, calculus disease, bladder cancer, sexual dysfunction including infertility, and the destroyed bladder and urethra. The management of filling bladder pressures and regular, complete emptying, ideally with clean intermittent catheterization, can prevent or delay many of these complications. Even with optimum management, complications may still develop over time, necessitating regular urologic follow-up to recognize, treat, and prevent further complications. The ultimate goal of the urologist in treating the patient with a neurogenic bladder is to allow for preservation of renal function and continence with minimum complications.

Index **609**

GOAL STATEMENT

The goal of *Urologic Clinics of North America* is to keep practicing urologists and urology residents up to date with current clinical practice in urology by providing timely articles reviewing the state of the art in patient care.

ACCREDITATION

The *Urologic Clinics of North America* is planned and implemented in accordance with the Essential Areas and Policies of the Accreditation Council for Continuing Medical Education (ACCME) through the joint sponsorship of the University of Virginia School of Medicine and Elsevier. The University of Virginia School of Medicine is accredited by the ACCME to provide continuing medical education for physicians.

The University of Virginia School of Medicine designates this educational activity for a maximum of 15 *AMA PRA Category 1 Credits*™ for each issue, 60 credits per year. Physicians should only claim credit commensurate with the extent of their participation in the activity.

The American Medical Association has determined that physicians not licensed in the US who participate in this CME activity are eligible for a maximum of 15 *AMA PRA Category 1 Credits*™ for each issue, 60 credits per year.

Credit can be earned by reading the text material, taking the CME examination online at http://www.theclinics.com/home/cme, and completing the evaluation. After taking the test, you will be required to review any and all incorrect answers. Following completion of the test and evaluation, your credit will be awarded and you may print your certificate.

FACULTY DISCLOSURE/CONFLICT OF INTEREST

The University of Virginia School of Medicine, as an ACCME accredited provider, endorses and strives to comply with the Accreditation Council for Continuing Medical Education (ACCME) Standards of Commercial Support, Commonwealth of Virginia statutes, University of Virginia policies and procedures, and associated federal and private regulations and guidelines on the need for disclosure and monitoring of proprietary and financial interests that may affect the scientific integrity and balance of content delivered in continuing medical education activities under our auspices.

The University of Virginia School of Medicine requires that all CME activities accredited through this institution be developed independently and be scientifically rigorous, balanced and objective in the presentation/discussion of its content, theories and practices.

All authors/editors participating in an accredited CME activity are expected to disclose to the readers relevant financial relationships with commercial entities occurring within the past 12 months (such as grants or research support, employee, consultant, stock holder, member of speakers bureau, etc.). The University of Virginia School of Medicine will employ appropriate mechanisms to resolve potential conflicts of interest to maintain the standards of fair and balanced education to the reader. Questions about specific strategies can be directed to the Office of Continuing Medical Education, University of Virginia School of Medicine, Charlottesville, Virginia.

The faculty and staff of the University of Virginia Office of Continuing Medical Education have no financial affiliations to disclose.

The authors/editors listed below have identified no professional or financial affiliations for themselves or their spouse/partner

Don T. Bui, MD; Frank N. Burks, MD; Anne P. Cameron, MD, FRCPS(C); Sung Yong Cho, MD; E. Ann Gormley, MD; Kerry Holland, (Acquisitions Editor); Seong Jin Jeong, MD; Edward J. McGuire, MD (Guest Editor); Majid Mirzazadeh, MD; Seung-June Oh, MD; Benjamin T. Ristau, MD; Marc C. Smaldone, MD; Irina Stanasel, MD; and John T. Stoffel, MD (Guest Editor).

The authors/editors listed below identified the following professional or financial affiliations for themselves or their spouse/partner

J. Quentin Clemens, MD, MSCI is a consultant for Pfizer, Lilly, Medtronic, and Afferent Pharmaceuticals; is an industry funded research/investigator for Pfizer; and owns stock in Merck.

Catherine Dalton, MRCPI is employed by the UCL, Institute of Neurology, London, through a grant from Novartis to perform MRI analysis in clinical trials for Multiple Sclerosis.

Clare J Fowler, FRCP is an industry funded research/investigator for Allergan and Astratech, and is on the Speakers' Bureau for Astellas, Medtronic, and Astratech.

Wendy W. Leng, MD is an industry funded research/investigator for Allergan.

Arthur Mourtzinos, MD is on the Speakers' Bureau for Pfizer, and is a consultant for Coloplast, American Medical Systems, and Ethicon.

Jalesh N. Panicker, MD, DM, MRCP (UK) is on the Speakers' Bureau for GSK and Sanofi Aventis.

Kenneth M. Peters, MD is an industry funded research/investigator for Boston Scientific, Cook Myosite, Uroplasty, J&J, Pfizer, and Allergan; is a consultant for Medtronic and Uroplasty; and is on the Advisory Committee/Board for Uroplasty.

John J. Smith III, MD is a research/consultant for Coloplast.

William Steers, MD (Test Author) is employed by the American Urologic Association, is a reviewer and consultant for NIH, and is an investigator for Allergan.

O. Lenaine Westney, MD is a consultant for American Medical Systems, and is employed as an investigator by Coloplast Corporation.

Disclosure of Discussion of Non-FDA Approved Uses for Pharmaceutical Products and/or Medical Devices.

The University of Virginia School of Medicine, as an ACCME provider, requires that all faculty presenters identify and disclose any off-label uses for pharmaceutical and medical device products. The University of Virginia School of Medicine recommends that each physician fully review all the available data on new products or procedures prior to clinical use.

TO ENROLL

To enroll in the Urologic Clinics of North America Continuing Medical Education program, call customer service at 1-800-654-2452 or visit us online at www.theclinics.com/home/cme. The CME program is available to subscribers for an additional fee of $207.00.

Urologic Clinics of North America

FORTHCOMING ISSUES

February 2011

Male Pelvic Health
Steven Kaplan, MD,
Guest Editor

May 2011

Erectile Dysfunction
Culley C. Carson, MD,
Guest Editor

August 2011

Complementary and Alternative Medicine in Urology
Mark A. Moyad, MD,
Guest Editor

RECENT ISSUES

August 2010

Penile and Urethral Cancer
Jack H. Mydlo, MD, FACS,
Guest Editor

May 2010

Pediatric Urology
Thomas F. Kolon, MD, FAAP,
Guest Editor

February 2010

Advances and Controversies in Prostate Cancer
William K. Oh, MD, and
Jim C. Hu, MD, MPH,
Guest Editors

Preface

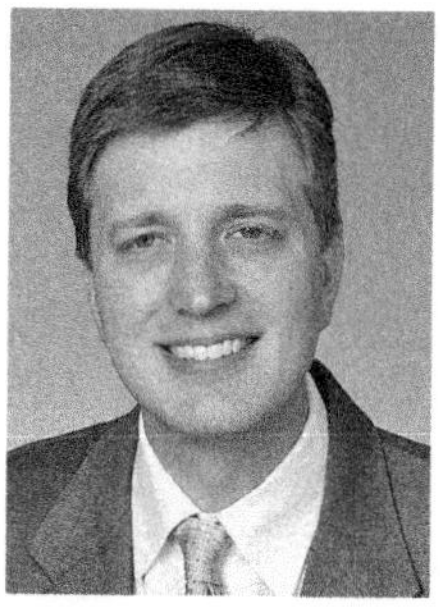
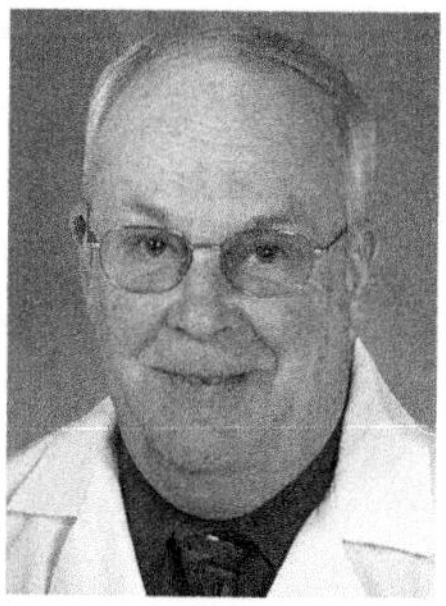

John T. Stoffel, MD   Edward J. McGuire, MD
Guest Editors

The term "neurogenic bladder" is broadly defined as any bladder disorder that is caused, or related to, an existing neurologic condition. Most urologists encounter a patient with a neurogenic bladder condition in daily practice. It is estimated that there are between 250,000 and 450,000 people living with spinal cord injuries in the United States and another 250,000–350,000 people who have been diagnosed with multiple sclerosis. Worldwide, more than 50 million people may be affected by neurologic conditions, such as spina bifida. Many patients with these, and other neurologic conditions, are now surviving longer due to improved treatments and are seeking urologic care for a myriad of urinary symptoms.

However, despite the homogenous definition, neurological conditions do not cause uniform bladder pathology. Some conditions will cause failure to store urine; others cause failure to empty urine, and unfortunately many conditions will result in both failure to store and failure to empty. To complicate matters further, the patient's urinary-specific quality of life may not always predict beneficial long-term health. Consequently, management of these patients can be challenging because there is no single best treatment for a neurogenic bladder.

Although preventing pathology requires patience and vigilance, understanding basic principles of managing the neurogenic bladder can directly improve both the length and the quality of these patients' lives. Rather than a single intervention, treatment of these patients is best thought of as a series of questions. To begin, urologists should seek to understand how the condition has affected the basic neurophysiology between the bladder, spinal cord, and brain. Once this physiology is better defined, treatment plans can be attempted so that urine is stored under stable low pressures and the bladder can be emptied with minimal residual. Next, urologists should ask how the condition may change over time and consequently affect the bladder. For example, patients with stable spinal cord injuries may need different follow-up compared to patients with secondarily progressive multiple sclerosis. Finally, urologists should constantly question if a different treatment would serve the patient better. Physicians should investigate the potential benefits and risks of established therapies, such as medications and surgery, and evolving treatments, such as neuromodulation and botulinium toxin, for the individual patient and have frequent discussion regarding options.

In this issue of *Urologic Clinics of North America*, our outstanding authors present current data on contemporary neurogenic bladder management principles. It is our hope that practicing urologists will apply many of these principles in the everyday care of his/her neurogenic bladder patient.

In the rapidly evolving world of neurophysiology, updated information on bladder signaling pathways and neurologic regulation of continence is presented. The ability and limitations surrounding urodynamics for defining pathophysiology are likewise considered. Regarding the natural history of neurologic conditions, progressive diseases such as Parkinson's disease, multiple system atrophy, and multiple sclerosis are reviewed from a urologic perspective. Management goals for spina bifida adults are proposed and data from spinal cord/vascular injured neurogenic bladder patients,

Urol Clin N Am 37 (2010) xi–xii
doi:10.1016/j.ucl.2010.07.005

including a meta-analysis of lesion and expected urologic symptom, are presented.

Contemporary treatment strategies are rapidly evolving and both established and cutting-edge future therapies are detailed. Goals and limitations of pharmacologic therapies are explained and potential new medications such as beta-adrenergic agonists and intravesical vanilloids are reviewed. The existing data on the efficacy of botulinum toxin in the neurogenic bladder are also objectively examined. Outcome data for urinary diversion in neurogenic bladder patients are described and novel applications, such as neuromodulation and tissue engineering, are proposed as potential future therapies. Finally, a review on managing and preventing urologic complications related to the neurogenic bladder serves as both a guide and a warning for urologists caring for these patients.

John T. Stoffel, MD
Department of Urology
Lahey Clinic, 41 Mall Road
Burlington, MA 01805, USA

Edward J. McGuire, MD
Department of Urology
University of Michigan School of Medicine
1500 East Medical Center Drive
Ann Arbor, MI 48109, USA

E-mail addresses:
john_t_stoffel@lahey.org (J.T. Stoffel)
edmcj@med.umich.edu (E.J. McGuire)

Basic Bladder Neurophysiology

J. Quentin Clemens, MD, MSCI

KEYWORDS

• Neuroanatomy • Physiology • Lower urinary tract
• Pharmacology

Normal lower urinary tract function requires the storage of urine at low intravesical pressure, without leakage. Intermittently, this storage function is interrupted by the voluntary and complete expulsion of urine. These processes (storage and voiding) are unique in that they involve the coordination of the peripheral autonomic, peripheral somatic, and central nervous systems (CNS). This article provides an overview of the basic principles that are recognized to regulate these functions, although many of these processes remain poorly understood. Furthermore, much of this knowledge has been obtained from in vivo animal models, and the relevance of these findings to human physiology is not always clear.

BLADDER ANATOMY AND BIOMECHANICS

The bladder base refers to the trigone and bladder neck, whereas the body consists of the supratrigonal portion.[1] The bladder wall consists (from the outside, away from the bladder lumen) of the serosa, smooth muscle and extracellular matrix (ECM) (in approximately 50-50 distribution), the lamina propria, and the urothelium. Like other smooth muscles, the detrusor muscle is oriented in a seemingly random fashion, is not attached to tendon or bone, is able to maintain steady tension over a wide range of muscle lengths, and has a slower contraction velocity than the skeletal muscle.[2,3] The detrusor muscle uses the ECM as a scaffold to generate tension, which produces a bladder contraction.

Bladder accommodation refers to the changes that occur during bladder filling to permit low-pressure urine storage across a wide range of bladder volumes. This process is measured by calculating the bladder compliance (change in bladder volume/change in intravesical pressure), which is expressed in mL/cm H_2O. Normal compliance is maintained throughout filling by reorientation of the detrusor smooth muscle fibers and connective tissue so that they are parallel to the lumen, thinning of the lamina propria, and flattening of the urothelium.[4] Bladder accommodation is a complex and poorly understood process that can be altered because of neurologic damage or changes in the ECM content. For instance, an increase in type III collagen has been found in bladders with decreased compliance.[5]

GENERAL NEUROANATOMY

The CNS consists of the brain and spinal cord, and the peripheral nervous system (PNS) consists of the sensory (afferent) and motor (efferent) neurons that communicate with the CNS. The PNS is divided into the somatic and the autonomic nervous systems. The somatic nervous system is responsible for regulating structures that are under conscious control (such as the striated external urethral sphincter and the levator muscles in the pelvic floor). The autonomic nervous system controls visceral and endocrine functions, including bladder contraction and relaxation. The autonomic nervous system is subdivided into the parasympathetic and sympathetic nervous systems. Sympathetic and parasympathetic are anatomic terms that indicate the location from where the nerve fibers emanate. Parasympathetic

Disclosures: Merck, stock ownership; Pfizer, consultant, investigator; Lilly, consultant; Afferent Pharmaceuticals, consultant; Medtronic, proctor.

Division of Neurourology and Pelvic Reconstructive Surgery, Department of Urology, University of Michigan Medical Center, 1500 East Medical Center Drive, Taubman Center 3875, Ann Arbor, MI 48109-5330, USA
E-mail address: qclemens@umich.edu

Urol Clin N Am 37 (2010) 487–494
doi:10.1016/j.ucl.2010.06.006
0094-0143/10/$ – see front matter

fibers emerge from the cranial and sacral segments of the spinal cord, whereas sympathetic fibers emerge from the thoracic and lumbar segments of the spinal cord.

CROSS-SECTIONAL ANATOMY OF THE SPINAL CORD

Peripheral sensory information is carried via afferent nerves fibers, which enter the dorsal (posterior) aspect of the spinal cord and then travel upward to the central processing centers in the CNS (**Fig. 1**). Afferent cell bodies are located in the dorsal root ganglia. The white matter of the spinal cord contains bundles of myelin-coated neurons, whereas the gray matter contains the cell bodies of interneurons and efferent motor neurons. Within the gray matter, nerve cell bodies are generally organized into functional clusters called nuclei (such as Onuf nucleus). Axons within the white matter are functionally grouped into tracts. Efferent motor axons exit from the ventral root of the spinal cord.

RELEVANT NEUROANATOMY: PNS AND SPINAL CORD

Preganglionic parasympathetic efferent nerves exit from the sacral segment of the spinal cord at S2 through S4. The axons travel a long distance within the pelvic nerve to the ganglia (pelvic plexus) that are located immediately adjacent to the end organ (bladder) (**Fig. 2**). These fibers modulate bladder contractions. The primary neurotransmitter for both pre- and postganglionic parasympathetic fibers is acetylcholine (ACh).[6]

Preganglionic sympathetic efferent nerves exit from the thoracolumbar segment of the spinal cord at T10 through L2. The ganglia for these nerves have variable locations: some are next to the vertebrae (paraganglia), some are between the vertebrae and the target organ (preganglia), and some are located with the end organ (peripheral ganglia).[7] Sympathetic efferent nerves to the lower urinary tract are located within the hypogastric nerve. The sympathetic efferent nerves modulate contractions of the urethral smooth muscle and bladder outlet and inhibit parasympathetic activity that promotes bladder contraction. The primary neurotransmitter for postganglionic sympathetic fibers is norepinephrine, but the primary neurotransmitter for preganglionic sympathetic fibers is ACh.

Preganglionic somatic efferent nerves exit from the sacral segment of the spinal cord at S2 through S4. Nerve bodies for these nerves are located in the Onuf nucleus, along the lateral border of the ventral gray matter in the sacral region of the spinal cord. The nerve fibers travel within the pudendal nerve to the external urethral sphincter, where they modulate striated (voluntary) sphincter contraction.[8]

In humans and animals, afferent nerves have been identified in the detrusor muscle and the suburothelium.[9,10] The suburothelial afferent nerve fibers form a plexus that lies immediately beneath the urothelial lining, with some nerve terminals extending into the urothelium itself. This plexus is more prominent in the trigone and bladder neck and relatively sparse in the bladder dome. Afferent nerve fibers from the lower urinary tract travel within the pelvic, hypogastric, and pudendal

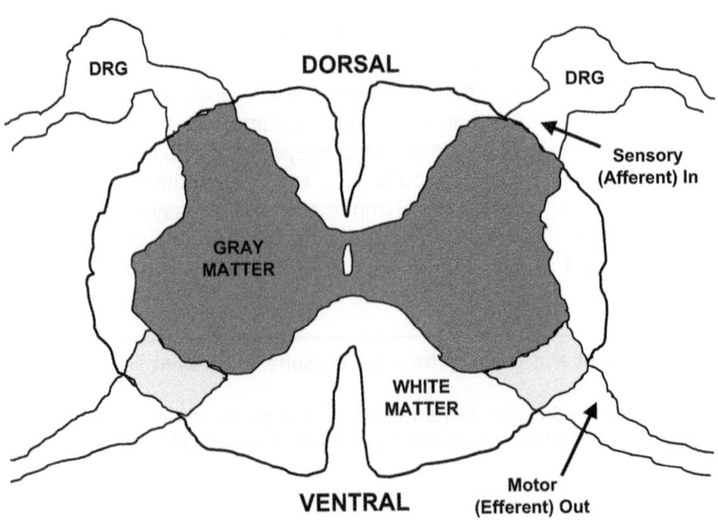

Fig. 1. Cross section of the sacral segment of the spinal cord. Sensory nerve fibers enter the dorsal spinal cord. Cell bodies of these sensory nerves are located in the dorsal root ganglia (DRG). The white matter contains bundles of neurons, whereas the gray matter contains the cell bodies of interneurons and efferent motor neurons. Motor nerve fibers exit the ventral spinal cord in the ventral root.

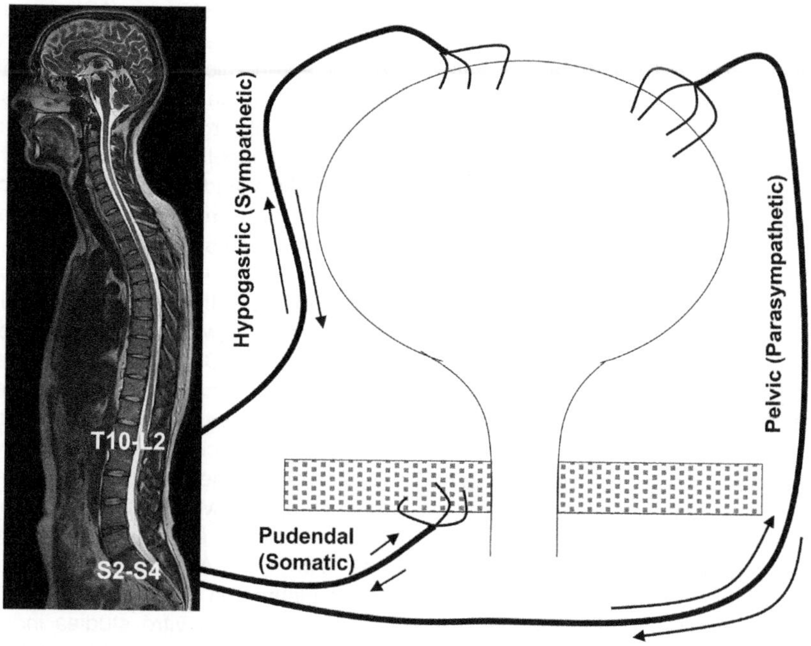

Fig. 2. Parasympathetic efferent nerves exit from the sacral region of the spinal cord at S2 through S4 and travel within the pelvic nerve. Parasympathetic activity promotes bladder emptying by causing contraction of the detrusor and relaxation of the bladder outlet. Sympathetic efferent nerves exit from the thoracolumbar segment of the spinal cord at T10 through L2 and travel within the hypogastric nerve. These nerves modulate contractions of the urethral smooth muscle and bladder outlet and inhibit parasympathetic activity that promotes bladder contraction. Somatic efferent nerves exit from the sacral segment of the spinal cord at S2 through S4 and travel within the pudendal nerve to the external urethral sphincter, where they modulate striated (voluntary) sphincter contraction. Afferent nerve fibers from the lower urinary tract travel within the pelvic, hypogastric, and pudendal nerves. Therefore, these peripheral nerves carry bidirectional (afferent and efferent) information between the end organs and the spinal cord.

nerves.[11,12] Therefore, these peripheral nerves carry bidirectional (afferent and efferent) information between the end organs and the spinal cord. The sensory fibers enter the spinal cord via the dorsal root, and the nerve cells bodies are located within the dorsal root ganglia. Afferent nerves release numerous neurotransmitters (eg, substance P, neurokinins, calcitonin gene–related polypeptide, vasoactive intestinal polypeptide).[13] Most sensory innervation of the bladder and urethra originates in the thoracolumbar region of the spinal cord and travels within the pelvic nerve.[12] Within the pelvic nerve, 2 types of bladder afferent nerves have been identified, myelinated Aδ fibers and unmyelinated C fibers. The Aδ fibers respond to normal bladder distention and are thought to be the primary functional afferent nerves during normal micturition.[12] Conversely, the C fibers respond to chemical irritation (nociception) or to cold, and most of these fibers are inactive during normal micturition.[14,15] However, during certain pathologic states (eg, inflammation, suprasacral spinal cord injury), these "silent" C fibers appear to activate, become mechanosensitive, and modulate pathologic voiding reflexes.[16]

RELEVANT NEUROANATOMY: BRAINSTEM AND ABOVE

Conclusive experimental evidence using brain-lesioning techniques, electric stimulation, and axonal tracing studies indicate that an area of the pons (the pontine micturition center [PMC] or Barrington nucleus) mediates the normal micturition reflex by coordinating the activity of the detrusor and urethral sphincter muscles.[17–20] Therefore, spinal cord lesions below this level often result in discoordination between the detrusor and urethral sphincter (detrusor-sphincter dyssynergia). The PMC receives input from multiple higher brain centers, including the basal ganglia, periaqueductal gray, thalamus, and hypothalamus.[21] Brain imaging studies in healthy volunteers suggest a model of supraspinal bladder control, in which afferent signals from the lower urinary tract are received in the periaqueductal gray and relayed via the thalamus to the insula (which makes the sensations accessible to conscious awareness).[22] According to this model, the cortex (via the anterior cingulate gyrus) monitors and controls micturition reflexes and also makes voluntary voiding decisions (via the prefrontal cortex).

NEURAL CONTROL OF THE LOWER URINARY TRACT

During the storage phase of micturition, bladder filling activates myelinated Aδ afferent nerve fibers in the bladder wall. This afferent input results in stimulation of sympathetic efferent activity (via the hypogastric nerve), leading to contraction of smooth muscles in the bladder base and proximal urethra (via activation of α-adrenergic receptors) and relaxation of the detrusor (via activation of β-adrenergic receptors in the bladder body). Somatic efferent activity (via the pudendal nerve) also increases, resulting in increased tone of the striated external urethral sphincter. These responses occur by spinal reflex pathways organized in the lumbosacral region of the spinal cord and represent guarding reflexes, which promote continence.[23–25] The parasympathetic system is largely inactive during urine storage, which may partly be because of the sympathetic inhibition of parasympathetic transmission at the ganglia level.

The voiding phase of micturition is initiated voluntarily by signals from the cerebral cortex. The initial event is relaxation of the striated external urethral sphincter, caused by inhibition of somatic efferent activity. There is inhibition of sympathetic efferent activity, with concomitant activation of parasympathetic outflow to the bladder and urethra.[26] Bladder contraction is mediated via muscarinic receptors in the bladder body, and urethral smooth muscle relaxation is mediated through the release of nitric oxide (NO).[27] Maintenance of the voiding reflex is a complicated phenomenon that is mediated via communication between the spinal cord and the pons (spinobulbospinal reflex), with the involvement of midbrain structures such as the periaqueductal gray.[21]

PHARMACOLOGY OF THE LOWER URINARY TRACT

Cholinergic Mechanisms

In certain neurons of the CNS and PNS, the neurotransmitter ACh is synthesized from the essential nutrient choline by the enzyme choline acetyltransferase. In response to various stimuli, ACh is released into the synaptic cleft, where it either binds to cholinergic receptors or is broken down by acetylcholinesterase. ACh is released from postganglionic parasympathetic neurons, preganglionic autonomic neurons (sympathetic and parasympathetic), and somatic neurons. Two main types of cholinergic receptors exist: nicotinic and muscarinic. Nicotinic receptors (which are responsive to ACh and nicotine) are ligand-gated ion channels and are found on the skeletal muscle motor end plates, on the autonomic ganglia, and in the CNS. The nicotinic receptors seem to have a limited role in the control of micturition. Muscarinic receptors (which are responsive to ACh and muscarine) are G protein–coupled receptors that activate ion channels via second-messenger cascades. These receptors are found on all autonomic effector cells (eg, bladder, sweat glands, bowel) and in the CNS. Five subtypes of muscarinic receptors (M_1 through M_5) have been identified, and the M_2 and M_3 subtypes predominate in the bladder.[28] Although M_2 receptors are the most plentiful in the detrusor (70% M_2 vs 30% M_3 receptors), in vitro studies indicate that the M_3 receptors are responsible for detrusor muscle contraction.[29–32] The functions of the detrusor M_2 receptors are less clear. Muscarinic receptors are also found on presynaptic nerve terminals in the bladder and elsewhere, where they may play a regulatory role via feedback inhibition.[33,34]

Excitation-contraction Coupling

Excitation-contraction coupling refers to the process whereby binding of a ligand to a receptor causes force generation (muscle contraction) (**Fig. 3**).[35] In the detrusor smooth muscle, the ligand is ACh and the receptor is the M_3 receptor. At rest, there is a very low concentration of free calcium ions (Ca^{2+}) in the smooth muscle cell. Binding of ACh to the M_3 receptor triggers a G protein–mediated process, which causes Ca^{2+} release from the sarcoplasmic reticulum as well as Ca^{2+} influx from transmembrane ion channels. The free Ca^{2+} binds to calmodulin, and the Ca^{2+}-calmodulin complex then activates the enzyme myosin light chain kinase, which phosphorylates the light chain of the contractile protein, myosin. This phosphorylation causes the myosin light chain to change shape and interact with actin, causing force generation.[35] Alongside this process, alternate methods are at work to facilitate subsequent muscle relaxation. The Ca^{2+}-calmodulin complex activates transmembrane Ca^{2+} pumps to remove free Ca^{2+} from the cell, the ligand-receptor complex is degraded, and excess extracellular ACh is degraded by acetylcholinesterase. This enzyme is abundant in the synaptic cleft, and its role in rapidly clearing free ACh

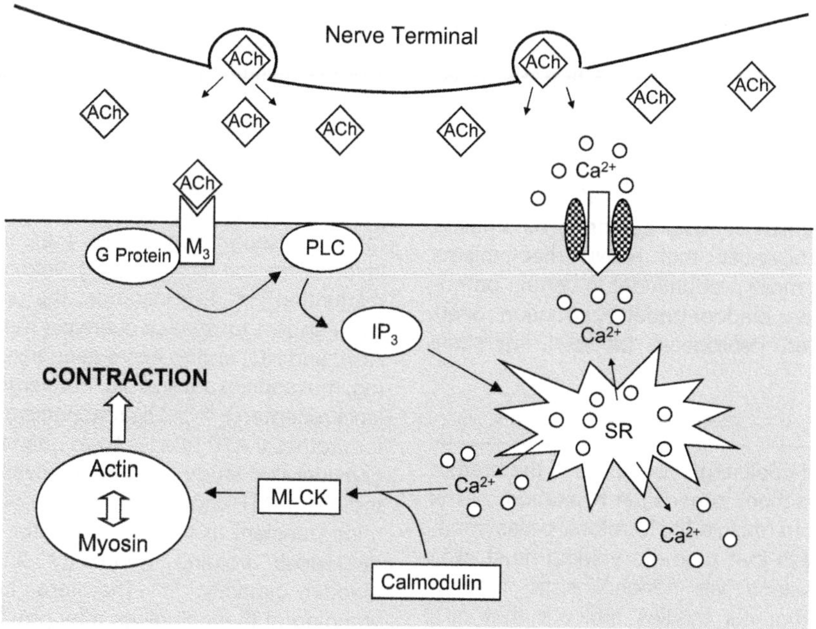

Fig. 3. Excitation-contraction coupling. Ach is released from postganglionic parasympathetic nerve terminals into the synaptic cleft, where it binds to the M_3 receptor. This ligand-receptor complex triggers a cascade of signaling events that involves a G protein, phospholipase C (PLC), and inositol triphosphate (IP_3). This signaling cascade leads to the release of free calcium (Ca^{2+}) into the cytosol by the sarcoplasmic reticulum (SR) as well as a direct influx of Ca^{2+} via transmembrane ion channels. The free Ca^{2+} binds with calmodulin, and the resulting Ca^{2+}-calmodulin complex activates the enzyme myosin light chain kinase (MLCK). The MLCK causes changes in the structure of the myosin molecule, which allows the myosin to interact with actin, leading to a muscle contraction.

from the synapse is essential for proper muscle function.

Adrenergic Mechanisms

Adrenergic receptors are G protein–coupled receptors that bind catecholamines (most commonly norepinephrine and epinephrine) that are released from postganglionic sympathetic neurons. Stimulation of α-adrenergic receptors causes vasoconstriction and smooth muscle contraction, whereas stimulation of β-adrenergic receptors causes increased myocardial contractility and smooth muscle relaxation. There exists multiple subtypes of adrenergic receptors. α-Adrenergic receptors were initially divided into α_1 (postsynaptic) and α_2 (presynaptic) receptors, but α_2 receptors were subsequently also found in postsynaptic locations. There are 3 subtypes of α_1 receptors (α_{1A}, α_{1B}, and α_{1D}). The α_{1A} subtype is the primary subtype in the prostate and urethra, where it mediates contraction of the bladder outlet.[36,37] The role of α_2 receptors in the lower urinary tract is not clear. There are 3 subtypes of β-adrenergic receptors (β_1, β_2, and β_3). β_1 Receptors are located in the heart, whereas β_2 and β_3 receptors are located in the lower urinary tract, where they cause detrusor smooth muscle relaxation.[38]

Receptor Distribution in the Lower Urinary Tract

The actions of the various neurotransmitters on the lower urinary tract are largely a function of receptor location.[39,40] There is a higher density of muscarinic receptors in the bladder body than in the base, and therefore activation of these receptors results in detrusor contraction. Adrenergic receptors are distributed such that α-adrenergic receptors (muscle contraction) predominate in the bladder base and urethra, whereas β-adrenergic receptors (muscle relaxation) predominate in the bladder body. Therefore, activation of the sympathetic nervous system promotes urine storage (relaxation of the bladder body and contraction of the outlet).

Nonadrenergic Noncholinergic Mechanisms of Bladder Excitation

In various mammalian species, complete blockage of cholinergic receptors with atropine does not pre-vent detrusor muscle contraction,[27] indicating that nonadrenergic noncholinergic (NANC) mechanisms exist, which at least partially mediate bladder contractions. In these nonhuman mammals, there is good evidence that the transmitter responsible for the NANC component of detrusor contraction is adenosine triphosphate (ATP) acting on purinergic receptors.[41,42] However, the component of NANC activation in the normal human detrusor seems to be small. It is possible, however, that NANC mechanisms may become more predominant in certain pathologic states (eg, bladder outlet obstruction, overactive bladder, neurogenic bladder, interstitial cystitis).[43,44]

Nitric Oxide

Stimulation of cholinergic receptors in the urethra causes contraction, rather than relaxation, of the urethral smooth muscle.[45] Therefore, parasympathetic pathways that promote voiding must elicit urethral relaxation via noncholinergic mechanisms. Experimental studies indicate that NO, released from postganglionic parasympathetic nerves, is the major inhibitory neurotransmitter that causes the urethral smooth muscle relaxation during voiding.[46,47] The mechanism of relaxation is similar to that observed in corporal smooth muscle (increased production of intracellular cyclic guanosine monophosphate and so forth). The functional role of NO in the detrusor has not been established.

Vanilloids

Vanilloids are a class of compounds denoted by the presence of a vanillyl functional group. Two vanilloids (capsaicin and resiniferatoxin [RTX]) are known to bind to receptors on C-fiber afferent neurons. This binding causes desensitization, so that the neurons no longer respond to stimuli. As discussed previously, C-fiber afferent neurons are considered to mediate pathologic bladder reflexes. Therefore, intravesical treatment with capsaicin and RTX has been examined as a potential therapy for conditions such as neurogenic detrusor overactivity and interstitial cystitis.[48,49]

Additional Neurotransmitters and Receptors

Multiple additional neurotransmitters and their associated receptors have been found to be synthesized, stored, and released in the human lower urinary tract, including tachykinins (eg, substance P, neurokinins), prostanoids (prostaglandins and thromboxanes), and endothelins.[13,35] However, the functional roles of most of these agents have not been established, and animal experiments suggest that these roles may vary across species.

SENSORY ROLE OF THE UROTHELIUM

The urothelium has traditionally been viewed as a passive barrier that prevents passage of urinary toxins into the underlying bladder interstitium. However, there is increasing evidence that the urothelium also has sensory and signaling properties that allow it communicate with nearby nerve and muscle tissue, suggesting that it is actively involved in the storage and voiding phases of micturition.[50,51] For instance, the urothelium has been shown to release chemical mediators (ATP, ACh, and NO) and to express numerous receptors (eg, muscarinic, adrenergic, purinergic, and tachykinin receptors).[35,52] The mechanisms responsible for urothelial ATP release have been the subject of considerable study because intravesical administration of ATP induces detrusor overactivity and mice deficient in the ATP receptor P2X3 exhibit decreased voiding frequency and increased bladder capacity.[53,54] Therefore, further understanding of these findings may provide additional therapeutic targets for lower urinary tract disorders.

REFERENCES

1. Elbadawi A, Schenk EA. Dual innervation of the mammalian urinary bladder, a histochemical study of the distributions of cholinergic and adrenergic nerves. Am J Anat 1966;119:405–27.
2. Uvelius B. Length-tension relations of in vitro urinary bladder smooth muscle strips. J Pharmacol Toxicol Methods 2001;45:87–90.
3. Uvelius B, Gabella G. Relation between cell length and force production in urinary bladder smooth muscle. Acta Physiol Scand 1980;110:357–65.
4. Chang SL, Chung JS, Yeung MK, et al. Roles of the lamina propria and the detrusor in tension transfer during bladder filling. Scand J Urol Nephrol Suppl 1999;201:38–45.
5. Landau EH, Jayanthi VR, Churchill BM, et al. Loss of elasticity in dysfunctional bladders: urodynamic and histochemical correlation. J Urol 1994;152:702–5.
6. de Groat WC, Booth AM. Synaptic transmission in pelvic ganglia. In: Maggi CA, editor. Nervous control of the urogenital system: the autonomic nervous system, vol. 3. London: Harwood Academic; 1993. p. 291–347.
7. Kihara K, de Groat WC. Sympathetic efferent pathways projecting to the bladder neck and proximal urethra in the rat. J Auton Nerv Syst 1997;62: 134–42.
8. Thor KB, Morgan C, Nadelhaft I, et al. Organization of afferent and efferent pathways in the pudendal nerve of the female cat. J Comp Neurol 1989;288: 263–79.

9. Dixon JS, Gilpin CJ. Presumptive sensory axons of the human urinary bladder: a fine structural study. J Anat 1987;151:199–207.
10. Gabella G, Davis C. Distribution of afferent axons in the bladder of rats. J Neurocytol 1998;27:141–55.
11. Yoshimura N, de Groat WC. Neural control of the lower urinary tract. Int J Urol 1997;4:111–25.
12. Janig W, Morrison JFB. Functional properties of spinal visceral afferents supplying abdominal and pelvic organs, with special emphasis on visceral nociception. Prog Brain Res 1986;67:87–114.
13. Andersson KE. Bladder activation: afferent mechanisms. Urology 2002;59(Suppl 5A):43–50.
14. Habler HJ, Janig W, Koltzenburg M. Activation of unmyelinated afferent fibres by mechanical stimuli and inflammation of the urinary bladder in the cat. J Physiol 1990;425:545–62.
15. Fall M, Lindstrom S, Mazieres L. A bladder-to-bladder cooling reflex in the cat. J Physiol 1990; 427:281–300.
16. de Groat WC, Kawatani M, Hisamitsu T, et al. Mechanisms underlying the recovery of urinary bladder function following spinal cord injury. J Auton Nerv Syst 1990;30:S71–7.
17. Barrington FJ. The effects of lesions of the hind and midbrain on micturition in the cat. Q J Exp Physiol 1925;15:81–102.
18. Mallory BS, Roppolo JR, de Groat WC. Pharmacologic modulation of the pontine micturition center. Brain Res 1991;546:310–20.
19. Holstege G, Griffiths D, De Wall H, et al. Anatomical and physiological observations on supraspinal control of the bladder and urethral sphincter muscles in the cat. J Comp Neurol 1986;250: 449–61.
20. Nadelhaft I, Vera PL, Card JP, et al. Central nervous system neurons labeled following the injection of pseudorabies virus into the rat urinary bladder. Neurosci Lett 1992;143:271–4.
21. Fowler CJ, Griffiths G, de Groat WC. The neural control of micturition. Nat Rev Neurosci 2008;9: 453–66.
22. Griffiths D, Tadic SD. Bladder control, urgency, and urge incontinence: evidence from functional brain imaging. Neurourol Urodyn 2008;27:466–74.
23. de Groat WC, Booth AM, Yoshimura N. Neurophysiology of micturition and its modification in animal models of human disease. In: Maggi CA, editor. Nervous control of the urogenital system: the autonomic nervous system, vol. 3. London: Harwood Acadmeic Publishers; 1993. p. 227.
24. de Groat WC, Vizzard MA, Araki I, et al. Spinal interneurons and preganglionic neurons in sacral autonomic reflex pathways. Prog Brain Res 1996;107: 97–111.
25. Park JM, Bloom DA, McGuire EJ. The guarding reflex revisited. Br J Urol 1997;80:940–5.
26. de Groat WC. Organization of the sacral parasympathetic reflex pathways to the urinary bladder and large intestine. J Auton Nerv Syst 1981;3:135–60.
27. Andersson KE. Pharmacology of lower urinary tract smooth muscles and penile erectile tissues. Pharmacol Rev 1993;45:253–308.
28. Bschleipfer T, Schukowski K, Weidner W, et al. Expression and distribution of cholinergic receptors in the human urothelium. Life Sci 2007;80:2303–7.
29. Harriss DR, Marsh KA, Birmingham AT, et al. Expression of muscarinic M3 receptors coupled to inositol phospholipid hydrolysis in human detrusor smooth muscle cells. J Urol 1995;154:1241–5.
30. Yamaguchi O, Shishido K, Tamura K, et al. Evaluation of mRNAs encoding muscarinic receptor subtypes in human detrusor muscle. J Urol 1996;156:1208–13.
31. Hegde SS, Choppin A, Bonhaus D, et al. Functional role of M2 and M3 muscarinic receptors in the urinary bladder of rats in vitro and in vivo. Br J Pharmacol 1997;120:1409–18.
32. Lai FM, Cobuzzi A, Spinelli W. Characterization of muscarinic receptors mediating the contraction of the urinary detrusor muscle in cynomolgus monkeys and guinea pigs. Life Sci 1998;62:1179–86.
33. D'Agostino G, Bolognesi ML, Lucchelli A, et al. Prejunctional muscarinic inhibitory control of acetylcholine release in the human isolated detrusor: involvement of the M4 receptor subtype. Br J Pharmacol 2000;129:493–500.
34. Somogyi GT, de Groat WC. Evidence for inhibitory nicotinic and facilitatory muscarinic receptors in cholinergic nerve terminals of the rat urinary bladder. J Auton Nerv Syst 1992;37:89–97.
35. Andersson KE, Arner A. Urinary bladder contraction and relaxation: physiology and pathophysiology. Physiol Rev 2004;84:935–86.
36. Furuya S, Kumamoto Y, Yokoyama E, et al. Alpha-adrenergic activity and urethral pressure in prostatic zone in benign prostatic hypertrophy. J Urol 1982; 128:836–9.
37. Nasu K, Moriyama N, Fukasawa R, et al. Quantification and distribution of alpha-1 adrenoreceptor subtype mRNAs in human proximal urethra. Br J Pharmacol 1998;123:1289–93.
38. Yamaguchi O. Beta 3-adrenoceptors in human detrusor muscle. Urology 2002;59(Suppl 1):25–9.
39. Johns A. Alpha- and beta-adrenergic and muscarinic cholinergic binding sites in the bladder and urethra of the rabbit. Can J Physiol Pharmacol 1983;61:61–6.
40. Levin RM, Ruggieri MR, Wein AJ. Identification of receptor subtypes in the rabbit and human urinary bladder by selective radio-ligand binding. J Urol 1988;139:844–8.
41. Lee HY, Bardini M, Burnstock G. Distribution of P2X receptors in the urinary bladder and the ureter of the rat. J Urol 2000;163:2002–7.

42. O'Reilly BA, Kosaka AH, Chang TK, et al. A quantitative analysis of purinoceptor expression in human fetal and adult bladders. J Urol 2001; 165:1730–4.
43. Bayliss M, Wu C, Newgreen D, et al. A quantitative study of atropine-resistant contractile responses in human detrusor smooth muscle from stable, unstable and obstructed bladders. J Urol 1999;162:1833–9.
44. Palea S, Artibani W, Ostardo E, et al. Evidence for purinergic neurotransmission in human urinary bladder affected by interstitial cystitis. J Urol 1993; 150:2007–12.
45. Ek A. Innervation and receptor functions of the human urethra. Scand J Urol Nephrol Suppl 1977; 45:1–50.
46. Andersson KE, Garcia Pascual A, Persson K, et al. Electrically-induced, nerve-mediated relaxation of rabbit urethra involves nitric oxide. J Urol 1992; 147:253–9.
47. Bennett BC, Kruse MN, Roppolo JR, et al. Neural control of urethral outlet activity in vivo: role of nitric oxide. J Urol 1995;153:2004–9.
48. Fowler CJ, Beck R, Gerrard S, et al. Intravesical capsaicin for treatment of detrusor hyperreflexia. J Neurol Neurosurg Psychiatry 1994;57: 169–73.
49. Payne CK, Mosbaugh PG, Forrest JB, et al. Intravesical resiniferatoxin for the treatment of interstitial cystitis: a randomized, double-blind, placebo controlled trial. J Urol 2005;173:1590–4.
50. Apodaca G. The uroepithelium: not just a passive barrier. Traffic 2004;5:117–28.
51. Ferguson DR. Urothelial function. BJU Int 1999;84: 235–42.
52. Birder LA, de Groat WC. Mechanisms of disease involvement of the urothelium in bladder dysfunction. Nat Clin Pract Urol 2007;4:46–54.
53. Pandita RK, Andersson KE. Intravesical ATP stimulates the micturition reflex in awake, freely moving rats. J Urol 2002;168:1230–4.
54. Cockayne DA, Hamilton SG, Zhu QM, et al. Urinary bladder hyporeflexia and reduced pain-related behaviour in P2X3-deficient mice. Nature 2000; 407:1011–5.

Pharmacologic Therapy for the Neurogenic Bladder

Anne P. Cameron, MD, FRCPS(C)

KEYWORDS

- Neurogenic urinary bladder • Muscarinic antagonists
- Alpha-adrenergic antagonist • Imipramine
- Spinal cord injury • Multiple sclerosis

Neurogenic bladder (NGB) is a heterogeneous diagnosis broadly describing bladder dysfunction because of neurologic insult. The symptoms range from urgency, frequency, and/or urgency incontinence to complete urinary retention, and the presentation is often different for the various causes. Diseases that are almost always associated with NGB include those with more severe neurologic dysfunction: spinal cord injury (SCI), multiple sclerosis (MS), and spina bifida; hence, these are the focus of this review. The goals of bladder management in NGB are the same, regardless of the cause. These goals are preservation of renal function, social continence, and efficient bladder emptying, which are achieved by treating most individuals in a targeted fashion based on urodynamic findings. The exception to this is MS, in which elevated bladder pressures[1] or upper tract damage are rare; therefore, symptoms and postvoid residuals (PVRs) are often sufficient to guide management.[2] NGB for other causes, such as diabetes, Parkinson disease, and rare neurologic disorders, has been less well studied; however, the general principles of bladder management in NGB would also apply to these disorders.

Bladder storage pressures ideally must be kept below 40 cm H_2O, because higher pressures carry a high risk of renal dysfunction and vesicoureteric reflux (VUR).[3] Bladder compliance must be maximized, because it is known that compliance less than or equal to 12.5 cm H20/ml often results in upper tract deterioration on radiological examination, VUR, and pyelonephritis.[4] Detrusor overactivity must also be treated, because it results in incontinence or increased pressure on the upper tract if there is detrusor sphincter dyssynergia (DSD).

Several oral and intravesical pharmacotherapeutic agents have been evaluated for treating detrusor overactivity and diminished bladder compliance in the NGB. These agents are the focus of this review, with surgical therapy and botulinum toxin injections being the subject of other articles in this series.

ANTICHOLINERGICS

Antimuscarinic (aka anticholinergic) medications have been the mainstay of pharmacologic therapy for neurogenic detrusor overactivity (NDO) for more than 30 years.[5] They decrease detrusor overactivity and significantly increase bladder capacity, reduce bladder filling pressure, improve compliance, reduce urge urinary incontinence events, and help to protect the upper urinary tract from deterioration.[6–8] Muscarinic receptor antagonists have traditionally been seen to act by binding to receptors on the detrusor muscle and thereby preventing acetylcholine release from parasympathetic nerves. These receptors are now known to be located on the detrusor and the mucosa,[9] and the newer pharmacotherapeutic

Funding: none.
Conflict of interest: The author has nothing to disclose.
Department of Urology, University of Michigan, 3875 Taubman Center, 1500 East Medical Center Drive, Ann Arbor, MI 48109-5330, USA
E-mail address: annepell@med.umich.edu

Urol Clin N Am 37 (2010) 495–506
doi:10.1016/j.ucl.2010.06.004
0094-0143/10/$ – see front matter. Published by Elsevier Inc.

agents have been shown to bind to both these receptor sites.[10]

Antimuscarinic use is recommended in NGB by the European Association of Urology[11] and a UK consensus group on the treatment of MS patients.[2] Furthermore, in a survey of the membership of the Society for Urodynamics and Female Urology, 84% thought that antimuscarinics and clean intermittent catheterization (CIC) were the best option for bladder management in SCI with detrusor overactivity.[12] However, a Cochrane review on anticholinergics for urinary symptoms in MS could not find sufficient evidence to support their use[13] given the lack of randomized controlled trials, but there exists level 1b evidence[14] of their effectiveness in MS and they are widely used.[2,14]

The side effects of the antimuscarinic drugs include dry mouth, constipation, blurred vision, drowsiness, and dry skin and mucosa. Dry mouth is the most common side effect, but many individuals with neurologic disorders are already using medications that cause dry mouth; hence, they often are unaware of the change. Also, bowel constipation seems to be less problematic, because most individuals have concomitant neurogenic bowel and already use laxatives, suppositories, and manual defecation.[6,15,16] Urinary retention is possible in those who void spontaneously; hence, upward dose titration in those individuals should be done carefully and PVRs monitored.[2,15,17] Retention is obviously not problematic in those who use CIC, and higher doses can be used. Even in studies in which the doses of antimuscarinics are doubled, the side-effect profile remains minimal, with significant increases in effectiveness.[7,15,17] Efficacy may be further increased by using 2 different antimuscarinics to take advantage of their slightly different receptor profiles while keeping side effects low.[7] It has also been observed that in the NGB population, higher doses are required to be effective compared with the non-neurogenic population.[17]

There is ample basic science evidence to support antimuscarinic therapy in NGB. In the human, there exist 5 muscarinic receptor subtypes M1 to M5,[18] however only M2 and M3 subtypes exist in the bladder.[19] The density of muscarinic receptors and the bladder's sensitivity to muscarinic agents is greatest in the dome and decreases toward the base of the bladder, which allows for efficient emptying of the bladder.[20] Muscarinic receptor density is also increased along with an increase in the sensitivity to muscarinic agonists after denervation of the bladder.[21,22] M2 receptors outnumber M3 receptors 3:1,[19] but it is the M3 receptors that mediate bladder contractions, at least in vitro, in normal bladders.[23] M3 knockout mice have significantly diminished bladder contractions, but only male animals develop significant bladder distention.[24] Because these animals continue to have bladder contractions, there are other muscarinic acetylcholine receptor subtypes or other mediators that rescue these contractions.[24]

The contribution of the M2 receptors is controversial. In muscarinic receptor knockout mouse models, including M2 knockout, M3 knockout, and double M2/M3 knockout animals, there is evidence to support the M2 receptor contributing to bladder contraction by rescuing the muscarinic contractile response after inactivation of the M3 receptors and enhancing the M3 receptor-mediated contractions. Detection of M2 receptor function is difficult when M3 and M2 receptors are activated, possibly explaining the difficulty in determining the true function of the M2 receptor.[25]

In the NGB, there is significant bladder remodeling with new expression of many proteins,[26] raising the possibility that the M2 receptors change in their density, increase in responsiveness, or both. In the denervated rat bladder, there is a 60% increase in M2 receptor density, and these M2 receptors provide a contractile function that is normally mediated by only M3 in normal bladder.[22,27] In the human bladder with NGB, M2 receptors were found to mediate contractions in one study[28] but were found to play no part in bladder contractions in another.[21]

There are currently several antimuscarinics available, but there are few head-to-head comparison studies. The vast majority of publications have been related to the idiopathic overactive bladder population.[29] However, the receptor mechanism behind NDO and idiopathic detrusor overactivity are believed to be similar.

In a meta-analysis of antimuscarinic therapy for overactive bladder (OAB), the longer-acting formulations were found to be more effective and to have decreased side effects, but little evidence supports the use of one long-acting agent over another.[29] However, there seems to be a difference in the cognitive impact of these drugs, especially on memory.[30] The pathophysiology behind this side effect is believed to be related to the drug penetrating the blood-brain barrier.[31] In a review of the current literature, oxybutynin was consistently associated with cognitive deficits, and darifenacin caused no detectable impairment in cognition. There was insufficient evidence to draw conclusions about the other antimuscarinics. The drug-related decrease in cognition was unnoticed by the patients in these studies.[30] Most studies were performed on healthy individuals, but the NGB population may be more susceptible to the effects of drugs that cross the blood-brain barrier, because individuals with MS,[32] stroke,[33] and Parkinson diseases actually have an increase in permeability.

Oxybutynin has long been used in the treatment of NGB. It is a commonly used drug in children with NGB and has been shown to be safe and effective regardless of the preparation (syrup, tablet, extended-release tablets, transdermal) in this population.[34,35] Oxybutynin is a tertiary amine metabolized by the liver that has antimuscarinic, spasmolytic, and local anesthetic properties,[36] but the spasmolytic and local anesthetic effects on detrusor smooth muscle are 500-fold weaker than the muscarinic receptor blocking.[37]

Extended-release (ER) oxybutynin has significantly fewer side effects that the immediate release and should be used if possible.[29] In individuals with NGB, when the dosage of oxybutynin ER is titrated upwards based on symptoms, side effects, and urodynamics, even including individuals who void spontaneously, the dose most often chosen is 30 mg/d.[17,38] The side effects do not increase linearly with dosage as is the case with immediate release oxybutinin.[39] Recently, transdermal oxybutynin systems have been evaluated in individuals with SCI,[40] with the expected improvements in the number of CICs per day, urinary leakage, maximum cystometric capacity (MCC), and detrusor pressures seen in other studies of the oral preparation. The incidence of dry mouth was low at 8.3%, but skin reactions to the patch were high at 12.5%.

A common misconception is that individuals with NGB managed with indwelling catheters do not benefit from antimuscarinic therapy. In a retrospective review of individuals with SCI who had indwelling catheters with or without oxybutynin for a mean of 11.9 years, bladder compliance was significantly better in those using oxybutynin. Complications, including hydronephrosis and febrile urinary tract infections, were much less frequent in those taking the medication as well.[8]

Intravesical administration of oxybutynin is only easily accomplished in individuals who already catheterize, which is why the neurogenic population are ideal candidates. Intravesical oxybutynin is absorbed systemically from the bladder but has fewer metabolites generated because of the reduced first-pass metabolism. These metabolites result in dry mouth and other side effects.[36] Also, mucosal muscarinic receptors in the bladder are blocked by oxybutynin, which are probably responsible for the effectiveness of intravesical administration[41] as well as afferent C-fibers that are inactivated by its local anesthetic effects.[42] Intravesical oxybutynin has been shown to significantly improve continence and quality of life in NGB.[43] Increasing doses of oxybutynin instilled intravesically increases effectiveness without a significant increase in side effects[44] and can be safely combined with oral antimuscarinics with better effectiveness.[45] Intravesical oxybutynin is prepared by breaking up standard oral tablets and dissolving them in water or saline with additives as needed. If larger batches are prepared for convenience, saline or water with gentamicin as an additive are better than tap water, because these are stable at room temperature for 4 weeks.[46] Although effective, intravesical administration is time-consuming and with the increased tolerability of ER oral preparations, remains an infrequent route of administration.

Tolterodine is an antimuscarinic that is equipotent with oxybutynin in the bladder but has an 8-fold lower affinity for the muscarinic receptors of the salivary glands.[47] Tolterodine is available in immediate release (IR) and ER formats. In clinical trials in individuals with NGB, it is as effective as oxybutynin at improving symptoms but has less incidence of dry mouth.[48] Tolterodine does reduce the QT interval on electrocardiogram,[16] hence the maximum daily dose is 8 mg. In randomized double-blind placebo controlled trials, tolterodine has been shown to improve urodynamic variables as well as continence and voided volumes, with increased effectiveness at 4 mg compared with 2 mg in NGB.[16] Increasing the dosage from 4 mg/d to 8 mg/d if incontinence persists is safe and effective in most patients with NGB.[15] In patients with MS, compared with oxybutynin, in an interim analysis of the cognitive safety of this drug, tolterodine showed a trend toward fewer cognitive side effects.[49] Recently, tolterodine has been expanded in its use to the pediatric NGB population, with the IR, ER, and oral solution showing improvements in bladder symptoms with a good safety profile.[50,51]

Trospium chloride is a quaternary amine with atropinelike effects[52] that has been studied in the NGB population. Compared with oxybutynin, it has an equivalent increase in MCC and bladder compliance and decrease in bladder storage pressures, but with considerably less dry mouth.[52] Dose escalation in individuals with insufficient clinical response is warranted, with improvements in all parameters with minimal increase in side effects even at doses up to 135 mg/d.[53,54]

The newer antimuscarinics, darifenacin,[55] solifenacin,[56] and fesoteridine,[57] have not been evaluated in the NGB population.[11] However, given their favorable side-effect profiles and similarity to other antimuscarinics, they are probably effective in NGB, but further data in this population are needed.

Propiverine is an antimuscarinic with additional calcium channel modulating properties,[58] and it is available in Europe for the treatment of OAB and NDO but is not currently Food and Drug Administration-approved. It is only available in an IR formulation. Propiverine is well tolerated in children and adolescents with NGB,[59] and when compared with oxybutynin, it has similar improvements in urodynamic MCC. However, propiverine was associated with fewer adverse events, especially dry mouth, fewer dropouts, and more children achieving normal detrusor pressures of 40 cm H_2O or less.[58] In a randomized double-blind study comparing IR propiverine and IR oxybutynin in adults with NGB, there were equivalent improvements in capacity, compliance, and detrusor pressure but improved side-effect profile with propiverine.[6]

α-BLOCKERS

α-Blockers are widely used for the treatment of benign prostatic hyperplasia (BPH),[60] and they relieve the voiding symptoms and associated bladder storage symptoms of urgency, frequency, and nocturia.[61] Their utility in NGB is often overlooked, despite their favorable side-effect profile, and there is evidence to support their use in the treatment of poor compliance, emptying difficulty, and autonomic dysreflexia (AD). α-Blockers are recommended as a possible treatment for NGB by the Clinical Practice Guidelines for the Paralyzed Veterans of America.[62]

α_1-adrenergic blockers that are currently used include alfuzosin, terazosin, doxazosin, and tamsulosin.[60] The more commonly reported side effects of these medications are nasal congestion, abnormal ejaculation (especially with tamsulosin), and dizziness or postural hypotension that are more common with doxazosin and terazosin, which is why these 2 drugs require dose escalation.[60]

There are significant basic science data to support α-blockers as a therapeutic option in NGB. There are three α_1-adrenergic receptor (AR) subtypes in the human: α_1a, α_1b, and α_1d.[63] Based on human histochemical studies, it is well known that the prostate and trigone contain predominantly α_1a-AR messenger (m)RNA and protein[64] and that α_1-AR–mediated smooth muscle contractions from sympathetic nervous system stimulation is the dynamic component of obstruction in BPH.[65]

However, α_1-ARs are not just present in the prostate. The human bladder dome and bladder base contain α_1a receptors, but the urothelium only contains the mRNA encoding the receptor, not the expressed protein.[66] In contrast to rats, a commonly used animal model of the bladder, only 2 types of α_1-AR are present in the human detrusor muscle: α_1a and α_1d in a 2:1 proportion, whereas the rat has a 1:1:1 proportion of a, b, and d.[67] Hence, one must interpret animal studies with caution, and human tissue studies need to be performed before any conclusions about receptor distribution or function can be drawn.[63]

α_1a-ARs are present in human arteries,[63] and all 3 receptors are present in the spinal cord, with a predominance of α_1d.[68] It is plausible that these spinal receptors impact the bladder. In the bladder, the AR number increases significantly in the NGB when compared with the normal bladder.[69]

Doxazosin has also been shown to play a sensory role in the bladder. Adenosine triphosphate (ATP) is released by the bladder urothelium when stretched, which in turn acts as a sensory neurotransmitter[70] and binds to the suburothelial sensory nerve endings via P2X3 receptors. This action sends an afferent signal to the brain indicating fullness of the bladder. Bladders of those with interstitial cystitis and of those with BPH released significantly more ATP compared with normal controls. This increase in ATP release was eliminated with doxazosin, which may explain how it relieves irritative symptoms in these patients.[71]

There are many articles on the study of phenoxybenzamine and prazosin, nonselective adrenergic blockers, with successful results in the treatment of NGB to facilitate bladder storage function.[72,73] In none of these trials, however, was there improvement in the ability to empty the bladder.[73] The high side-effect profile of both drugs and the theoretical risk of malignancy with long-term usage of phenoxybenzamine has limited their use. Newer, more selective α_1-blockers are safer choices,[60] even in this population.[74,75]

Voiding is not possible in many individuals with NGB, and treatment with α-blockers does not appear to change this state.[73] However, in several studies of individuals with NGB who can spontaneously void with a residual volume, the newer α-blockers have been shown to be effective. In a study of 28 patients with DSD, American Urological Association symptom index, PVRs, and urodynamic urine flow all improved with 2 months of treatment with tamsulosin.[76] In a study of 24 patients with NGB examined with urodynamics before and after 1 month of 0.4 mg tamsulosin, there were no changes in residual volume, but the maximum flow rate on free uroflow and the maximum detrusor pressure on urodynamics were improved after treatment.[74]

In a 4-week randomized controlled trial (RCT) of 263 patients with suprasacral SCI followed by a 1-year open label study of placebo compared with tamsulosin, maximum urethral pressure (MUP), the primary outcome of the study, was not significantly different between groups at the 4-week mark. However, in the 186 patients who completed the 1-year open label study, there were significant improvements in MUP (−18 cm H2O) as well as improved MCC, PVR, and voiding time. There were also improvements seen in incontinence and other lower urinary tract symptoms in the treated group. On a global assessment by the investigators, 71% of treated patients were improved on the 1-year follow-up study.[75]

Other investigators have also successfully demonstrated a dose-dependent reduction in MUP with intravenous alfuzosin in 163 patients with NGB.[77] Upper tract stasis on renal scan, presumably because of poor voiding in men with SCI of T6 and above who reflex-voided improved in 8 of 10 men started on α-blockers.[78]

There is evidence that α-blockers are also effective in MS for help in bladder emptying. In a placebo-controlled RCT of 18 men with MS younger than 50 years with elevated PVR, indoramin, an α_1-adrenergic blocker, improved flow by 41%. Seven-ninths of patients on the indoramin reported improvement in their symptoms and 4 had enough objective and subjective improvement to elect to continue the medication long-term.[79]

α-Blocker therapy has also been shown to improve AD symptoms in SCI individuals. Prazosin was shown to be effective in a group of 16 symptomatic patients compared with placebo,[80] but this drug is not currently used because of high systemic side effects. In prospective trials, terazosin, which is well tolerated in the SCI population, has been shown to reduce the frequency of AD episodes and the severity of the symptoms,[81] with only minor side effects of fatigue[82] and dizziness,[83] and it did not cause changes in resting blood pressure or impact erectile function.[81] In the aforementioned RCT of tamsulosin, Alzheimer disease symptoms were improved in those individuals with injuries above T6, with 44% becoming symptom-free.[75]

The impact of α-blockers on bladder storage symptoms, including capacity, compliance, and detrusor pressure, has been less well evaluated. Some authors have reported no change in capacity or compliance with urapidil, an α-blocker available in Europe,[84] but maximum detrusor pressures[74] and bladder capacity[75] have been improved in other studies on tamsulosin.

IMIPRAMINE

Tricyclic antidepressants (TCAs), in particular imipramine, have been shown to suppress bladder overactivity by various mechanisms. Imipramine. a muscarinic receptor agonist, directly inhibits smooth muscle[85] and decreases bladder overactivity by blocking the reuptake of serotonin.[86] Other effects include the peripheral blockade of noradrenaline, stimulating the β-receptors at the dome of the bladder, which in turn decreases bladder contractility.[87] In clinical trials, imipramine has been shown to increase compliance in the pediatric NGB[88,89] and to improve incontinence in adults with NGB.[90] To date, TCAs have no RCTs to support their use for urologic indications and have been related to cardiac events, so must be used with caution, especially in the elderly. Imipramine, however, has been one of the major pharmacotherapeutic strategies to treat nocturnal enuresis, with success rates of 40% to 70%.[91,92]

COMBINATION THERAPY

There is evidence that α-blockers act in a synergistic fashion when combined with antimuscarinic therapy. The rationale for dual therapy is that by blocking different bladder receptors, effectiveness is increased and the side-effect profile of the two therapies at physiologic doses is theoretically better than simply increasing the antimuscarinic therapy. This combination is also safe and frequently used to treat refractory storage symptoms in men with BPH who have failed α-blocker therapy on its own.[93]

In an SCI primate model, intravenous antimuscarinics improved urodynamic bladder compliance compared with placebo. When phenoxybenzamine, an α-blocker, was added to the antimuscarinic, the compliance was further improved, indicating that α-blockers impact the bladder independent of voiding function.[94] In a clinical study of 12 individuals with SCI who had poor bladder compliance despite taking an antimuscarinic and performing CIC, the addition of 5 mg of terazosin for 1 month significantly improved their bladder capacity, pressures, and compliance. These urodynamic improvements disappeared after stopping the α-blocker, indicating the reversibility of their action.[95]

Other combination therapies that have been successful and safely used include tricyclic antidepressants in combination with anticholinergics in children with nocturnal enuresis that was resistant to TCAs alone.[96]

Two independent studies have reported their results in treating individuals with refractory incontinence or poor compliance because of NGB with triple drug therapy, consisting of an antimuscarinic combined with an α-blocker and imipramine.[97,98] In this group of individuals who were refractory to antimuscarinics alone, maximum detrusor pressure, capacity, and bladder compliance were all improved as was the resolution of subjective patient incontinence. Side effects were tolerable, the most common being dry mouth and constipation.[99]

OTHER THERAPIES ON THE HORIZON

In preliminary studies on the SCI rat, 48 genes have already been identified that are significantly upregulated in their expression after traumatic SCI. Their functions include carbohydrate, lipid, histamine, amino acid, androgen, and estrogen metabolism. This illustrates the significant gene expression changes that occur to cause the clinically observed bladder remodeling.[26] Given the large number of alterations that occur in the bladder after SCI, it is inevitable that future research will unveil new therapeutic targets. Several of these targets that have significant promise have been studied and may provide the next generation of pharmacotherapy for NGB detrusor overactivity.

The human bladder contains 3 β-ARs (β_1, β_2, and β_3), with 97% of the β-receptors being β_3.[99] Selective β_3-receptor agonists relax detrusor muscle, and β_3-adrenoceptor activation is the main method of bladder relaxation.[100] Therefore, these are an ideal target for the treatment of detrusor overactivity.[99] There are currently phase II and III clinical trials underway for the treatment of OAB using these promising therapies.[101]

Another therapeutic option in intravesical therapies that has shown great promise are capsaicin (CAP) and resiniferatoxin (RTX). These agents have activity on vanilloid receptors located on afferent nerves in the bladder that are mainly small unmyelinated C fibers. These agents act differently, in that CAP initially depolarizes then blocks or desensitizes the C fiber, whereas RTX is an ultrapotent analog that is 1000 times more potent for desensitization and hundreds of times more potent for excitation.[102] One must recall that C fibers normally carry only the response to noxious stimuli and seem to have a limited role in normal voiding. However, after SCI, it seems that C fibers become sensitive to bladder filling, not just noxious stimuli. This leads to a new C-fiber–mediated voiding reflex that plays a major part in spinal detrusor hyperreflexia.[103]

Many studies have used CAP diluted in a 30% ethanol solution and have reported poor tolerability of this agent,[104] but when one compared 30% ethanol to CAP dissolved in 30% ethanol, the side effects of suprapubic pain, hematuria, and detrusor overactivity are the same, indicating that the concentrated alcohol is the likely culprit.[105] In a trial comparing CAP to RTX, with the CAP diluted in a glucidic solvent instead of 30% alcohol, there were equivalent clinical and urodynamic improvements seen in a group of individuals with SCI and NDO, with these benefits remaining in two-thirds of individuals at 90 days with equivalent side effects in the 2 groups.[104] However, a systematic review of neurotoxins in NGB and a recent RCT concluded that botulinum toxin type A injections are superior to resiniferatoxin.[106,107]

The bladder body contracts in the presence of ATP, whereas the base of the bladder does not.[20] ATP signals via P2X1 receptors and participates in the efferent control of detrusor muscle contractions. ATP is significantly more potent at generating bladder contractions in the diseased bladder compared with normal. ATP is also involved in bladder sensations via the P2X2 and P2X2/3 receptors on sensory afferent neurons within the bladder itself.[108] Purinergic receptors (P2X2) are found in normal bladders, but are overexpressed in human SCI.[109] Currently, several agents target the purinergic receptors as a potential drug target.[108]

Other therapies that may show promise in the future include cannabinoids in the form of cannabis extract or Δ9-tetrahydrocannabinol. In an RCT, patients with MS showed significant improvements in urgency incontinence and pad weights but not urodynamics or quality of life compared with placebo.[110]

In the bladder, serotonin is believed to potentiate the cholinergic response. Serotonin (5-hydroxytryptamine) receptor blockers are a potential target for the treatment of NGB, although their potentiation is believed to be lower compared with that in normal bladders.[111] Clinically, paroxetine, a selective serotonin reuptake inhibitor, did not change urodynamic variables or voiding diaries in a group of individuals with NGB from various causes who all voided spontaneously, but milnacipran, a serotonin-norepinephrine reuptake inhibitor, did increase bladder capacity and decrease frequency.[112] Antiepileptic drugs have been shown to improve bladder function in animal[113] and human[114] studies of NGB. Other therapeutic targets that have shown promise thus far in animal models of NGB include cyclooxygenase inhibitor,[115] an

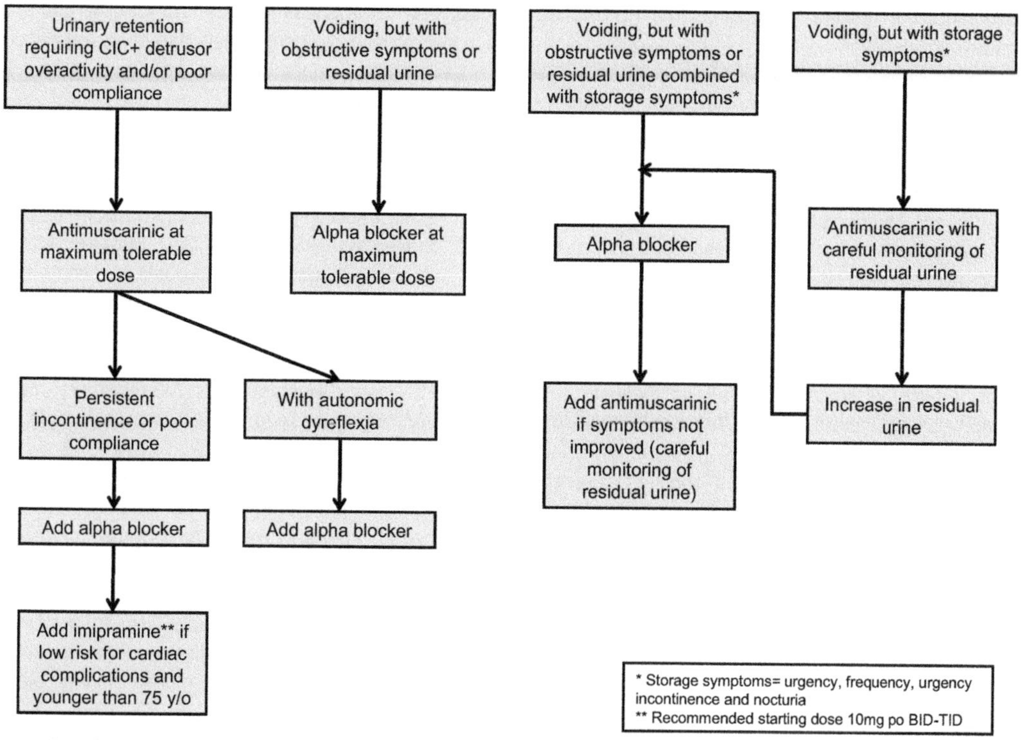

Fig. 1. Flowchart of pharmacologic treatment of neurogenic bladder based on symptoms and urodynamic findings.

arginase inhibitor,[116] endothelin-A receptor agonist,[117] and gene therapy with glutamic acid decarboxylase.[118]

SUMMARY

Antimuscarinic therapy is the mainstay in treatment for NGB with detrusor overactivity or poor compliance, with robust basic science and clinical data to support its use. α-Blockers have less evidence to guide their use in NGB but are safe medications with good evidence to support their effectiveness in NGB, particularly in individuals who are able to void. They can be used in combination with antimuscarinics to improve AD and bladder storage. In those who void, but with an elevated PVR or obstructive symptoms, antimuscarinic therapy can push someone into retention, hence treatment with an α-blocker, initially, can prevent this and improve voiding. Imipramine, although studied mostly in combination with the aforementioned drugs in triple drug therapy, has been shown to improve bladder compliance. Recommendations on the use of these therapies alone or in combination are outlined in **Fig. 1**.

Many therapeutic targets are under investigation and many more are yet to be discovered to aid in the management of NGB, and until stem cell research and other new therapies discover a method to reinnervate the bladder, there remains a great need.

REFERENCES

1. Lemack GE, Frohman E, Ramnarayan P. Women with voiding dysfunction secondary to bladder outlet dyssynergia in the setting of multiple sclerosis do not demonstrate significantly elevated intravesical pressures. Urology 2007;69(5):893–7.
2. Fowler CJ, Panicker JN, Drake M, et al. A UK consensus on the management of the bladder in multiple sclerosis. J Neurol Neurosurg Psychiatry 2009;80(5):470–7.
3. McGuire EJ, Woodside JR, Borden TA. Upper urinary tract deterioration in patients with myelodysplasia and detrusor hypertonia: a followup study. J Urol 1983;129(4):823–6.
4. Weld KJ, Graney MJ, Dmochowski RR. Differences in bladder compliance with time and associations of bladder management with compliance in spinal cord injured patients. J Urol 2000;163(4):1228–33.
5. Hebjorn S. Treatment of detrusor hyperreflexia in multiple sclerosis: a double-blind, crossover clinical trial comparing methantheline bromide (Banthine), flavoxate chloride (Urispas) and

meladrazine tartrate (Lisidonil). Urol Int 1977;32 (2–3):209–17.
6. Stohrer M, Murtz G, Kramer G, et al. Propiverine compared to oxybutynin in neurogenic detrusor overactivity–results of a randomized, double-blind, multicenter clinical study. Eur Urol 2007;51 (1):235–42.
7. Amend B, Hennenlotter J, Schafer T, et al. Effective treatment of neurogenic detrusor dysfunction by combined high-dosed antimuscarinics without increased side-effects. Eur Urol 2008;53(5): 1021–8.
8. Kim YH, Bird ET, Priebe M, et al. The role of oxybutynin in spinal cord injured patients with indwelling catheters. J Urol 1997;158(6):2083–6.
9. Bschleipfer T, Schukowski K, Weidner W, et al. Expression and distribution of cholinergic receptors in the human urothelium. Life Sci 2007;80 (24–25):2303–7.
10. Mansfield KJ, Chandran JJ, Vaux KJ, et al. Comparison of receptor binding characteristics of commonly used muscarinic antagonists in human bladder detrusor and mucosa. J Pharmacol Exp Ther 2009;328(3):893–9.
11. Stohrer M, Blok B, Castro-Diaz D, et al. EAU guidelines on neurogenic lower urinary tract dysfunction. Eur Urol 2009;56:81–8.
12. Razdan S, Leboeuf L, Meinbach DS, et al. Current practice patterns in the urologic surveillance and management of patients with spinal cord injury. Urology 2003;61(5):893–6.
13. Nicholas RS, Friede T, Hollis S, et al. Anticholinergics for urinary symptoms in multiple sclerosis. Cochrane Database Syst Rev 2009;1:CD004193
14. Gajewski JB, Awad SA. Oxybutynin versus propantheline in patients with multiple sclerosis and detrusor hyperreflexia. J Urol 1986;135(5):966–8.
15. Horstmann M, Schaefer T, Aguilar Y, et al. Neurogenic bladder treatment by doubling the recommended antimuscarinic dosage. Neurourol Urodyn 2006;25(5):441–5.
16. Van Kerrebroeck PE, Amarenco G, Thuroff JW, et al. Dose-ranging study of tolterodine in patients with detrusor hyperreflexia. Neurourol Urodyn 1998;17(5):499–512.
17. Bennett N, O'Leary M, Patel AS, et al. Can higher doses of oxybutynin improve efficacy in neurogenic bladder? J Urol 2004;171(2 Pt 1):749–51.
18. Caulfield MP, Birdsall NJ. International Union of Pharmacology. XVII. Classification of muscarinic acetylcholine receptors. Pharmacol Rev 1998;50 (2):279–90.
19. Wang P, Luthin GR, Ruggieri MR. Muscarinic acetylcholine receptor subtypes mediating urinary bladder contractility and coupling to GTP binding proteins. J Pharmacol Exp Ther 1995;273(2): 959–66.
20. Levin RM, Shofer FS, Wein AJ. Cholinergic, adrenergic and purinergic response of sequential strips of rabbit urinary bladder. J Pharmacol Exp Ther 1980;212(3):536–40.
21. Stevens LA, Chapple CR, Chess-Williams R. Human idiopathic and neurogenic overactive bladders and the role of M2 muscarinic receptors in contraction. Eur Urol 2007;52(2):531–8.
22. Braverman AS, Luthin GR, Ruggieri MR. M2 muscarinic receptor contributes to contraction of the denervated rat urinary bladder. Am J Physiol 1998;275(5 Pt 2):R1654–60.
23. Chess-Williams R, Chapple CR, Yamanishi T, et al. The minor population of M3-receptors mediate contraction of human detrusor muscle in vitro. J Auton Pharmacol 2001;21(5–6):243–8.
24. Matsui M, Motomura D, Karasawa H, et al. Multiple functional defects in peripheral autonomic organs in mice lacking muscarinic acetylcholine receptor gene for the M3 subtype. Proc Natl Acad Sci U S A 2000;97(17):9579–84.
25. Ehlert FJ, Griffin MT, Abe DM, et al. The M2 muscarinic receptor mediates contraction through indirect mechanisms in mouse urinary bladder. J Pharmacol Exp Ther 2005;313(1):368–78.
26. Tseng LH, Chen I, Lin YH, et al. Genome-based expression profiling study following spinal cord injury in the rat: an array of 48-gene model. Neurourol Urodyn 2010. [Epub ahead of print].
27. Braverman AS, Ruggieri MR. Selective alkylation of rat urinary bladder muscarinic receptors with 4-DAMP mustard reveals a contractile function for the M2 muscarinic receptor. J Recept Signal Transduct Res 1999;19(5):819–33.
28. Pontari MA, Braverman AS, Ruggieri MR. The M2 muscarinic receptor mediates in vitro bladder contractions from patients with neurogenic bladder dysfunction. Am J Physiol Regul Integr Comp Physiol 2004;286(5):R874–80.
29. Novara G, Galfano A, Secco S, et al. A systematic review and meta-analysis of randomized controlled trials with antimuscarinic drugs for overactive bladder. Eur Urol 2008;54(4):740–63.
30. Kay GG, Ebinger U. Preserving cognitive function for patients with overactive bladder: evidence for a differential effect with darifenacin. Int J Clin Pract 2008;62(11):1792–800.
31. Kay GG, Granville LJ. Antimuscarinic agents: implications and concerns in the management of overactive bladder in the elderly. Clin Ther 2005; 27(1):127–38, quiz 139–40.
32. Kwon EE, Prineas JW. Blood-brain barrier abnormalities in longstanding multiple sclerosis lesions. An immunohistochemical study. J Neuropathol Exp Neurol 1994;53(6):625–36.
33. Dietrich WD, Prado R, Halley M, et al. Microvascular and neuronal consequences of common

carotid artery thrombosis and platelet embolization in rats. J Neuropathol Exp Neurol 1993;52(4): 351–60.
34. Franco I, Horowitz M, Grady R, et al. Efficacy and safety of oxybutynin in children with detrusor hyperreflexia secondary to neurogenic bladder dysfunction. J Urol 2005;173(1):221–5.
35. Cartwright PC, Coplen DE, Kogan BA, et al. Efficacy and safety of transdermal and oral oxybutynin in children with neurogenic detrusor overactivity. J Urol 2009;182:1548–54.
36. Buyse G, Waldeck K, Verpoorten C, et al. Intravesical oxybutynin for neurogenic bladder dysfunction: less systemic side effects due to reduced first pass metabolism. J Urol 1998;160 (3 Pt 1):892–6.
37. Yarker YE, Goa KL, FittonOxybutynin A. A review of its pharmacodynamic and pharmacokinetic properties, and its therapeutic use in detrusor instability. Drugs Aging 1995;6(3):243–62.
38. O'Leary M, Erickson JR, Smith CP, et al. Effect of controlled-release oxybutynin on neurogenic bladder function in spinal cord injury. J Spinal Cord Med 2003;26(2):159–62.
39. Thuroff JW, Bunke B, Ebner A, et al. Randomized, double-blind, multicenter trial on treatment of frequency, urgency and incontinence related to detrusor hyperactivity: oxybutynin versus propantheline versus placebo. J Urol 1991;145(4):813–6 [discussion: 816–7].
40. Kennelly MJ, Lemack GE, Foote JE, et al. Efficacy and safety of oxybutynin transdermal system in spinal cord injury patients with neurogenic detrusor overactivity and incontinence: an open-label, dose-titration study. Urology 2009;74:741–5.
41. Kim Y, Yoshimura N, Masuda H, et al. Antimuscarinic agents exhibit local inhibitory effects on muscarinic receptors in bladder-afferent pathways. Urology 2005;65(2):238–42.
42. De Wachter S, Wyndaele JJ. Intravesical oxybutynin: a local anesthetic effect on bladder C afferents. J Urol 2003;169(5):1892–5.
43. Vaidyananthan S, Soni BM, Brown E, et al. Effect of intermittent urethral catheterization and oxybutynin bladder instillation on urinary continence status and quality of life in a selected group of spinal cord injury patients with neuropathic bladder dysfunction. Spinal Cord 1998; 36(6):409–14.
44. Haferkamp A, Staehler G, Gerner HJ, et al. Dosage escalation of intravesical oxybutynin in the treatment of neurogenic bladder patients. Spinal Cord 2000;38(4):250–4.
45. Pannek J, Sommerfeld HJ, Botel U, et al. Combined intravesical and oral oxybutynin chloride in adult patients with spinal cord injury. Urology 2000;55(3):358–62.
46. Wan J, Rickman C. The durability of intravesical oxybutynin solutions over time. J Urol 2007;178 (4 Pt 2):1768–70.
47. Nilvebrant L, Andersson KE, Gillberg PG, et al. Tolterodine–a new bladder-selective antimuscarinic agent. Eur J Pharmacol 1997;327(2–3):195–207.
48. Ethans KD, Nance PW, Bard RJ, et al. Efficacy and safety of tolterodine in people with neurogenic detrusor overactivity. J Spinal Cord Med 2004;27 (3):214–8.
49. Nagels G, De DEyn P, Vleugels L, et al. A prospective randomized double blind cross-over dose titration study to evaluate the cognitive safety profile of tolterodine as compared to oxybutynin in multiple sclerosis patients with overactive bladder: a planned interim analysis [abstract 237]. Presented at the Annual ICS meeting, 2004. Available at: https://www.icsoffice.org/ASPNET_Membership/Membership/Abstracts/AbstractsSearch.aspx?EventID=42. Accessed June 26, 2010.
50. Reddy PP, Borgstein NG, Nijman RJ, et al. Long-term efficacy and safety of tolterodine in children with neurogenic detrusor overactivity. J Pediatr Urol 2008;4(6):428–33.
51. Mahanta K, Medhi B, Kaur B, et al. Comparative efficacy and safety of extended-release and instant-release tolterodine in children with neural tube defects having cystometric abnormalities. J Pediatr Urol 2008;4(2):118–23.
52. Madersbacher H, Stohrer M, Richter R, et al. Trospium chloride versus oxybutynin: a randomized, double-blind, multicentre trial in the treatment of detrusor hyper-reflexia. Br J Urol 1995;75(4):452–6.
53. Madersbacher H, Stohrer M, Richter R, et al. High-dose trospium chloride in therapy of detrusor hyperreflexia. Urologe A 1991;30(4):260–3.
54. Menarini M, Del Popolo G, Di Benedetto P, et al. Trospium chloride in patients with neurogenic detrusor overactivity: is dose titration of benefit to the patients? Int J Clin Pharmacol Ther 2006;44 (12):623–32.
55. Chapple CR. Darifenacin: a novel M3 muscarinic selective receptor antagonist for the treatment of overactive bladder. Expert Opin Investig Drugs 2004;13(11):1493–500.
56. Oki T, Sato S, Miyata K, et al. Muscarinic receptor binding, plasma concentration and inhibition of salivation after oral administration of a novel antimuscarinic agent, solifenacin succinate in mice. Br J Pharmacol 2005;145(2):219–27.
57. Herschorn S, Swift S, Guan Z, et al. Comparison of fesoterodine and tolterodine extended release for the treatment of overactive bladder: a head-to-head placebo-controlled trial. BJU Int 2010; 105(1):58–66.
58. Madersbacher H, Murtz G, Alloussi S, et al. Propiverine vs oxybutynin for treating neurogenic

detrusor overactivity in children and adolescents: results of a multicentre observational cohort study. BJU Int 2009;103(6):776–81.
59. Grigoleit U, Murtz G, Laschke S, et al. Efficacy, tolerability and safety of propiverine hydrochloride in children and adolescents with congenital or traumatic neurogenic detrusor overactivity–a retrospective study. Eur Urol 2006;49(6):1114–20 [discussion: 1120–1].
60. Djavan B, Chapple C, Milani S, et al. State of the art on the efficacy and tolerability of alpha1-adrenoceptor antagonists in patients with lower urinary tract symptoms suggestive of benign prostatic hyperplasia. Urology 2004;64(6):1081–8.
61. Nordling J. Efficacy and safety of two doses (10 and 15 mg) of alfuzosin or tamsulosin (0.4 mg) once daily for treating symptomatic benign prostatic hyperplasia. BJU Int 2005;95(7):1006–12.
62. Consortium for Spinal Cord Medicine. Bladder management for adults with spinal cord injury: a clinical practice guideline for health-care providers. J Spinal Cord Med 2006;29(5):527–73.
63. Schwinn DA. Novel role for alpha1-adrenergic receptor subtypes in lower urinary tract symptoms. BJU Int 2000;86(Suppl 2):11–20 [discussion: 20–2].
64. Price DT, Schwinn DA, Lomasney JW, et al. Identification, quantification, and localization of mRNA for three distinct alpha 1 adrenergic receptor subtypes in human prostate. J Urol 1993;150(2 Pt 1):546–51.
65. Forray C, Bard JA, Wetzel JM, et al. The alpha 1-adrenergic receptor that mediates smooth muscle contraction in human prostate has the pharmacological properties of the cloned human alpha 1c subtype. Mol Pharmacol 1994;45(4):703–8.
66. Walden PD, Durkin MM, Lepor H, et al. Localization of mRNA and receptor binding sites for the alpha 1a-adrenoceptor subtype in the rat, monkey and human urinary bladder and prostate. J Urol 1997;157(3):1032–8.
67. Malloy BJ, Price DT, Price RR, et al. Alpha1-adrenergic receptor subtypes in human detrusor. J Urol 1998;160(3 Pt 1):937–43.
68. Smith MS, Schambra UB, Wilson KH, et al. Alpha1-adrenergic receptors in human spinal cord: specific localized expression of mRNA encoding alpha1-adrenergic receptor subtypes at four distinct levels. Brain Res Mol Brain Res 1999;63(2):254–61.
69. Restorick JM, Mundy AR. The density of cholinergic and alpha and beta adrenergic receptors in the normal and hyper-reflexic human detrusor. Br J Urol 1989;63(1):32–5.
70. Sun Y, Keay S, De Deyne PG, et al. Augmented stretch activated adenosine triphosphate release from bladder uroepithelial cells in patients with interstitial cystitis. J Urol 2001;166(5):1951–6.
71. Sun Y, MaLossi J, Jacobs SC, et al. Effect of doxazosin on stretch-activated adenosine triphosphate release in bladder urothelial cells from patients with benign prostatic hyperplasia. Urology 2002;60(2):351–6.
72. Kaplan PE, Nanninga JB. Reduction of bladder contractility after alpha-adrenergic blockade and after ganglionic blockade. Acta Neurol Scand 1979;59(4):172–7.
73. Petersen T, Husted SE, Sidenius P. Prazosin treatment of neurological patients with detrusor hyperreflexia and bladder emptying disability. Scand J Urol Nephrol 1989;23(3):189–94.
74. Kakizaki H, Ameda K, Kobayashi S, et al. Urodynamic effects of alpha1-blocker tamsulosin on voiding dysfunction in patients with neurogenic bladder. Int J Urol 2003;10(11):576–81.
75. Abrams P, Amarenco G, Bakke A, et al. Tamsulosin: efficacy and safety in patients with neurogenic lower urinary tract dysfunction due to suprasacral spinal cord injury. J Urol 2003;170(4 Pt 1):1242–51.
76. Stankovich EI, Borisov VV, Demina TL. [Tamsulosin in the treatment of detrusor-sphincter dyssynergia of the urinary bladder in patients with multiple sclerosis]. Urologiia 2004;4:48–51 [in Russian].
77. Perrigot M, Delauche-Cavallier MC, Amarenco G, et al. Effect of intravenous alfuzosin on urethral pressure in patients with neurogenic bladder dysfunction. DORALI Study Group. Neurourol Urodyn 1996;15(2):119–31.
78. Linsenmeyer TA, Horton J, Benevento J. Impact of alpha1-blockers in men with spinal cord injury and upper tract stasis. J Spinal Cord Med 2002;25(2):124–8.
79. O'Riordan JI, Doherty C, Javed M, et al. Do alpha-blockers have a role in lower urinary tract dysfunction in multiple sclerosis? J Urol 1995;153(4):1114–6.
80. Krum H, Louis WJ, Brown DJ, et al. A study of the alpha-1 adrenoceptor blocker prazosin in the prophylactic management of autonomic dysreflexia in high spinal cord injury patients. Clin Auton Res 1992;2(2):83–8.
81. Chancellor MB, Erhard MJ, Hirsch IH, et al. Prospective evaluation of terazosin for the treatment of autonomic dysreflexia. J Urol 1994;151(1):111–3.
82. Chancellor MB, Anderson RU, Boone TB. Pharmacotherapy for neurogenic detrusor overactivity. Am J Phys Med Rehabil 2006;85(6):536–45.
83. Vaidyanathan S, Soni BM, Sett P, et al. Pathophysiology of autonomic dysreflexia: long-term treatment with terazosin in adult and paediatric spinal cord injury patients manifesting recurrent

dysreflexic episodes. Spinal Cord 1998;36(11): 761–70.
84. Yasuda K, Yamanishi T, Kawabe K, et al. The effect of urapidil on neurogenic bladder: a placebo controlled double-blind study. J Urol 1996;156(3): 1125–30.
85. Levin RM, Staskin DR, Wein AJ. Analysis of the anticholinergic and musculotropic effects of desmethylimipramine on the rabbit urinary bladder. Urol Res 1983;11(6):259–62.
86. Maggi CA, Borsini F, Lecci A, et al. Effect of acute or chronic administration of imipramine on spinal and supraspinal micturition reflexes in rats. J Pharmacol Exp Ther 1989;248(1):278–85.
87. Hoebeke PB, Vande Walle J. The pharmacology of paediatric incontinence. BJU Int 2000;86(5):581–9.
88. Dave S, Grover VP, Agarwala S, et al. The role of imipramine therapy in bladder exstrophy after bladder neck reconstruction. BJU Int 2002;89(6): 557–60 [discussion: 560–1].
89. Puri A, Bhatnagar V, Grover VP, et al. Urodynamics-based evidence for the beneficial effect of imipramine on valve bladders in children. Eur J Pediatr Surg 2005;15(5):347–53.
90. Cole AT, Fried FA. Favorable experiences with imipramine in the treatment of neurogenic bladder. J Urol 1972;107(1):44–5.
91. Owens RG, Karram MM. Comparative tolerability of drug therapies used to treat incontinence and enuresis. Drug Saf 1998;19(2):123–39.
92. Smellie JM, McGrigor VS, Meadow SR, et al. Nocturnal enuresis: a placebo controlled trial of two antidepressant drugs. Arch Dis Child 1996;75 (1):62–6.
93. Kaplan SA, Roehrborn CG, Rovner ES, et al. Tolterodine and tamsulosin for treatment of men with lower urinary tract symptoms and overactive bladder: a randomized controlled trial. JAMA 2006;296(19):2319–28.
94. McGuire EJ, Savastano JA. Effect of Alpha-adrenergic blockade and anticholinergic agents on the decentralized primate bladder. Neurourol Urodyn 1985;4:139–42.
95. Swierzewski SJ. The effect of terazosin on bladder function in the spinal cord injured patient. J Urol 1994;151(4):951.
96. Kaneko K, Fujinaga S, Ohtomo Y, et al. Combined pharmacotherapy for nocturnal enuresis. Pediatr Nephrol 2001;16(8):662–4.
97. Cameron AP, Clemens JQ, Latini JM, et al. Combination drug therapy improves compliance of the neurogenic bladder. J Urol 2009;182(3):1062–7.
98. Natalin R, Reis LO, Alpendre C, et al. Triple therapy in refractory detrusor overactivity: a preliminary study. World J Urol 2010;28:79–85.
99. Yamaguchi O. Beta3-adrenoceptors in human detrusor muscle. Urology 2002;59(5 Suppl 1):25–9.
100. Biers SM, Reynard JM, Brading AF. The effects of a new selective beta3-adrenoceptor agonist (GW427353) on spontaneous activity and detrusor relaxation in human bladder. BJU Int 2006;98(6): 1310–4.
101. Drake MJ. Emerging drugs for treatment of overactive bladder and detrusor overactivity. Expert Opin Emerg Drugs 2008;13(3):431–46.
102. Szallasi A, Blumberg PM. Vanilloid receptors: new insights enhance potential as a therapeutic target. Pain 1996;68(2–3):195–208.
103. de Groat WC. Mechanisms underlying the recovery of lower urinary tract function following spinal cord injury. Paraplegia 1995;33(9):493–505.
104. de Seze M, Wiart L, de Seze MP, et al. Intravesical capsaicin versus resiniferatoxin for the treatment of detrusor hyperreflexia in spinal cord injured patients: a double-blind, randomized, controlled study. J Urol 2004;171(1):251–5.
105. de Seze M, Wiart L, Joseph PA, et al. Capsaicin and neurogenic detrusor hyperreflexia: a double-blind placebo-controlled study in 20 patients with spinal cord lesions. Neurourol Urodyn 1998;17(5): 513–23.
106. Giannantoni A, Di Stasi SM, Stephen RL, et al. Intravesical resiniferatoxin versus botulinum-A toxin injections for neurogenic detrusor overactivity: a prospective randomized study. J Urol 2004;172 (1):240–3.
107. MacDonald R, Monga M, Fink HA, et al. Neurotoxin treatments for urinary incontinence in subjects with spinal cord injury or multiple sclerosis: a systematic review of effectiveness and adverse effects. J Spinal Cord Med 2008;31(2):157–65.
108. Ford AP, Gever JR, Nunn PA, et al. Purinoceptors as therapeutic targets for lower urinary tract dysfunction. Br J Pharmacol 2006;147(Suppl 2): S132–43.
109. Pannek J, Janek S, Sommerer F, et al. Expression of purinergic P2X2-receptors in neurogenic bladder dysfunction due to spinal cord injury: a preliminary immunohistochemical study. Spinal Cord 2009;47(7):561–4.
110. Freeman RM, Adekanmi O, Waterfield MR, et al. The effect of cannabis on urge incontinence in patients with multiple sclerosis: a multicentre, randomised placebo-controlled trial (CAMS-LUTS). Int Urogynecol J Pelvic Floor Dysfunct 2006;17(6):636–41.
111. Chapple CR, Radley SC, Martin SW, et al. Serotonin-induced potentiation of cholinergic responses to electrical field stimulation in normal and neurogenic overactive human detrusor muscle. BJU Int 2004;93(4):599–604.
112. Sakakibara R, Ito T, Uchiyama T, et al. Effects of milnacipran and paroxetine on overactive bladder due to neurologic diseases: a urodynamic assessment. Urol Int 2008;81(3):335–9.

113. Elzayat EA, Campeau L, Karsenty G, et al. Effect of antiepileptic agent, levetiracetam, on urodynamic parameters and neurogenic bladder overactivity in chronically paraplegic rats. Urology 2009;73(4): 922–7.
114. Carbone A, Palleschi G, Conte A, et al. Gabapentin treatment of neurogenic overactive bladder. Clin Neuropharmacol 2006;29(4):206–14.
115. Tanaka I, Nagase K, Tanase K, et al. Improvement in neurogenic detrusor overactivity by peripheral C fiber's suppression with cyclooxygenase inhibitors. J Urol 2010;183(2):786–92.
116. Sasatomi K, Hiragata S, Miyazato M, et al. Nitric oxide-mediated suppression of detrusor overactivity by arginase inhibitor in rats with chronic spinal cord injury. Urology 2008;72(3):696–700.
117. Ogawa T, Sasatomi K, Hiragata S, et al. Therapeutic effects of endothelin-A receptor antagonist on bladder overactivity in rats with chronic spinal cord injury. Urology 2008;71(2):341–5.
118. Miyazato M, Sasatomi K, Hiragata S, et al. GABA receptor activation in the lumbosacral spinal cord decreases detrusor overactivity in spinal cord injured rats. J Urol 2008;179(3):1178–83.

Urodynamics of the Neurogenic Bladder

Edward J. McGuire, MD

KEYWORDS

• Urodynamics • Neurogenic bladder • Detrusor pressure
• Spinal cord injury • Myelodysplasia

HISTORICAL REVIEW

Identification of Risk Factors in Lower Urinary Tract Dysfunction Associated with Neurologic Lesions or Diseases

Spinal cord injuries

Before the 1970s and well into the1980s and beyond, risk factors associated with lower urinary tract dysfunction were not well established. The complications associated with neurogenic vesical dysfunction and obstructive uropathy were known, but the pathophysiology of these processes was not. What happened to most people with a neurogenic bladder was recognized and even expected, but knowledge of precisely why this happened was not. For example, Bors and Comarr[1] published a landmark textbook, *Neurologic Urology*, on the neurogenic bladder in 1971, which was the authoritative work in the field for many years. A good illustration of the prevailing concepts of treatment of the neurogenic bladder after spinal cord injury at the time of the book is the manner in which intermittent catheterization was used. The authors used sterile intermittent catheterization for the first 90 days after a spinal cord injury was incurred, as after that time, "90% of patients will have recovered bladder function."[1] This was based on the work on intermittent catheterization at the Stoke-Mandeville Rehabilitation Center in England. Recovery of reflex bladder function did not imply normalcy or even safety, because the cumulative risks of neurogenic urinary tract dysfunction continued to threaten most patients with spinal cord injury over time. However, the goal of short-term intermittent catheterization was to restore balanced bladder function and thus, a catheter-free state, implying an infection-free situation. Sterile intermittent catheterization was used to treat a spinal shock bladder with the expectation of recovery of reflex bladder activity. Balanced bladder function was defined by a residual urine volume 30% or less than bladder capacity. A considerable percentage of patients did briefly achieve balanced bladder function temporarily. Those who did not and most of those who did so transiently but failed to maintain that state were usually treated with indwelling catheters.

The authors noted that the progression of lower urinary tract disease was slow, and complications related to that process developed slowly in the first 5 years after spinal cord injury, then faster during the next 10 years. In parallel with the progression of lower urinary tract disease was a progressive loss of renal function. Factors identified in association with progressive urinary and renal dysfunction included chronic catheterization, vesicoureteral reflux, bladder spasticity, and urinary infection. Treatment was not specific and was largely reactive. For example, Foley catheters were used when balanced bladder function failed. These catheters were replaced by suprapubic tubes when bladder catheters failed and then by nephrostomy tubes or ileal loop diversion as the disease progressed. DeVivo and colleagues,[2] in 1993, noted that the death rate from sepsis in patients with spinal cord injury was 82 times the expected rate based on age. In addition to sepsis, the complications of neurogenic vesical dysfunction included and still include renal failure, hypertension, stone formation, incontinence, skin breakdown, tissue loss, osteomyelitis, dystrophic calcification, urethral erosion and destruction, autonomic dysreflexia, vesicoureteral reflux, and death. These complications were well known and seemingly not preventable. As an example of the

Department of Urology, University of Michigan School of Medicine, 1500 East Medical Center Drive, Ann Arbor, MI 48109, USA
E-mail address: edmcj@med.umich.edu

Urol Clin N Am 37 (2010) 507–516
doi:10.1016/j.ucl.2010.06.002
0094-0143/10/$ – see front matter

severity of the progressive urologic disease in patients with spinal cord injury, by 10 years after injury, most were managed by catheters. In these patients, there was a very high rate of fistula and abscess formation, a 70% calculus rate, and, with time, a very high rate of renal failure and bladder malignancy.[1]

Neurogenic bladder in children

In children with myelodysplasia, despite close observation in excellent centers, 48% developed upper tract complications by age 5 years as reported by Kasabian and coworkers[3] in 1992 and Wang and coworkers[4] in 1988. Those myelodysplastic children with very high-grade vesicoureteral reflux were often treated by cutaneous loop ureterostomy to decompress the upper urinary tracts as reported by Cass and Giest[5] in 1972. That surgery did decompress the upper urinary tract but it ignored the real problem, bladder storage pressures, which were the root cause of the ureteral obstruction, dilation, vesicoureteral reflux, and renal failure. Bauer and coworkers,[6] in 1982, reported on the management of vesicoureteral reflux in myelodysplasia. They used intermittent catheterization, cutaneous vesicostomy, and antireflux surgery. They had reasonable results, but it is clear from reading the paper that the underlying problem, detrusor pressure (Pdet), was not yet recognized. Sidi and coworkers,[7] in 1986, described their experience with 58 children with myelodysplasia, 52% of whom had vesicoureteral reflux. Of these, most responded to decompressive treatment, but 12 of 14 children with high-grade reflux required an antireflux operation. The investigators noted that in some children, upper tract changes and deterioration continued despite the surgery. Unlike children with reflux in the absence of a neurogenic bladder in whom operative intervention was nearly always successful, in myelodysplastic children, Pdet is the problem: a factor not influenced by antireflux surgery. By 2002, Simforoosh and coworkers[8] reported that ureteral reimplantation was not necessary in patients with neurogenic vesical dysfunction and vesicoureteral reflux undergoing augmentation cystoplasty, because control of Pdet achieved by the surgery eliminated vesicoureteral reflux. Conversely, Momose and coworkers,[9] in 1993, reported on 2 patients with neurogenic vesical dysfunction and vesicoureteral reflux who were judged unsuitable for augmentation cystoplasty and instead were treated by Cohen-type ureteral cross-trigonal reimplantation with predictable results; the reflux persisted as did the risk. In these children, reflux is pressure-driven and not the result of poor ureteral valve function.

Late treatment of complications related to management of the neurogenic bladder

In patients with spinal cord injury, myelodysplastic children, and patients with multiple sclerosis, ileal loop diversions or cutaneous ureterostomies are done to salvage a damaged urinary tract or, occasionally, as a prophylactic measure to prevent such damage. In either case, late outcomes for these procedures in patients with neurogenic vesical dysfunction are not good.

For example, Shapiro and coworkers,[10] in 1975, noted that although creatinine clearance remained normal over a 10-year period in most of their patients treated by ileal loop diversion, complications were serious and numerous. Cass and coworkers,[11] in 1984, reported a 22-year follow-up of children treated by ileal loop diversion. They noted that deterioration in the upper urinary tracts began to occur after 10 years in addition to a high earlier complication rate. Mitchell and coworkers[12] reported on ileal stenosis as a late complication of urinary diversion resulting in a fibrotic, noncompliant loop with a risk of renal failure. This report was amplified by Simeone and coworkers[13] in 2003.They described ileal loop stenosis as an insidious process (seen years after loop formation) of loop fibrosis, which is associated with upper tract damage. This problem, known at the University of Michigan Urology Department as old loop syndrome, can only be treated by creating a new loop. From departmental experience, this problem is seen beginning at 10 years after loop formation (Konnak J, personal communication, 2009).

Another late problem is parastomal hernia formation, which can be associated with loop obstruction, ureteral and renal damage, and bleeding from the stoma, among other problems.

Repair can be equally problematic. Pastor and coworkers[14] reported on 25 patients who underwent parastomal hernia repair and noted immediate complications in 6 patients and hernia recurrence in 11 patients (44%). Wan and colleagues,[15] in 1992, reported on 71 patients with neurogenic vesical dysfunction treated for upper urinary tract stones.

Patients with catheters or ileal loop diversions had the highest rate of stone formation and the most serious problems with stones and renal deterioration. In 1994, Breza and coworkers[16] reported on 6 patients aged 7 to 22 years after ileal loop diversion, who developed serious upper tract complications and required undiversion into a continent low-pressure reservoir with resulting stabilization of upper urinary tract function. Hetet and coworkers,[17] in 2005, reported on 246 patients who had an ileal loop diversion between January 1990 and December 2002. Mean follow-up was 24 months, and complications included fistula, evisceration, and ileus in 46 patients; medical complications resulted in 10 deaths; late urologic complications, including fistula, hernia, and peristomal hernia, occurred in 21% of patients and other urologic complications, including pyelonephritis, ureteral ileal stenosis and stones, in 21%. Although similar complications related to incontinent urinary diversion are not often reported in elderly patients undergoing ileal loop diversion as part of extirpative pelvic surgery for malignancy, these problems are time-related; as such, they are an important issue for younger patients who are diverted early on in the course of their neurologic disease, either prophylactically or as a way to deal with complications of managing their neurogenic bladder. Early prospective management guided by urodynamic testing can prevent urinary diversion.

Other methods of management of the neuropathic bladder

Through the late 70s and into the 80s, there were sporadic reports on the management of the spinal cord injury-affected bladder with a procedure to decrease outlet resistance. These procedures included external sphincterotomy, bladder neck incision, and transurethral resection of the proximal sphincter in men and women. In men, outlet procedures required condom catheters to control the resultant incontinence, but late outcomes were reasonable in the few series reporting late results.[18,19] Success was largely judged by a decrease in residual urine volumes, which was thought to be the major factor in urinary tract infection (UTI) and thus, risk. Most men with cervical spinal lesions did not achieve low residual urine volumes, and thus, repeated sphincterotomies were often required. For example, Whitmore and coworkers,[18] in 1978, described good short-term results with anteromedian sphincterotomy in spinal cord injured patients. Petri and coworkers,[19] in 1978, described bladder neck resection or incision in 86 adults with neurogenic vesical dysfunction and noted a good effect on flow, reflux, ureteral status, and infection rates. Continence is affected by these procedures , although they do reduce bladder pressure.

Movements away from prompt urinary drainage

In 1972, Lapides and colleagues[20] introduced clean intermittent catheterization as a short-term method of management of urinary retention associated with several urologic conditions. This technique would later be applied to patients with neurogenic vesical dysfunction from several causes. Lapides,[21] in 1979, thought that bladder overdistension induced bladder ischemia, thus exacerbating problems related to infection. If bladder volumes and pressures were kept low, infection would theoretically not be a problem. The early experience with intermittent catheterization in patients with retention was favorable. Although it is probably not absolutely true that simple freedom from bladder ischemia is the major advantage of intermittent catheterization, it quickly became clear that chronic bacteriuria did not produce wholesale death from sepsis in patients who managed their bladder with clean intermittent catheterization. That, in 1972 and 1979, was an astonishing revelation, because, for years, papers noted that pyelonephritis and renal failure could follow even a single catheterization. Last and coworkers,[22] in 1966, noted a relationship between urological instrumentation and bacteremia. Barton and coworkers,[23] in 1984, examined kidneys after death in patients with end-stage renal disease related to spinal cord injury and concluded that pathologic findings of amyloidosis, acute and chronic pyelonephritis, renal abscess formation, calculus disease, and pyelonephrosis were much more common in the patient population with spinal cord injury than in those without. They concluded that more effective treatment of urinary infections might help to alleviate end-stage renal disease in patients with spinal cord injury. That ideation persists today. Chronic bacterial colonization of the neurogenic bladder managed by clean intermittent catheterization or after augmentation cystoplasty is routinely treated with antibiotics, even though it is clear that eradication of chronic bacilluria in these cases never occurs.

In 1981, Kass and others[24] from the Lapides unit at Michigan University described their experience with intermittent catheterization in children with myelodysplasia. They noted that chronic bacteriuria was not a risk factor in patients without vesicoureteral reflux (VUR) or in those with low-grade VUR. Conversely, those children with high-grade reflux and chronic bacteriuria did develop progressive upper tract disease despite intermittent catheterization. The data and the concepts described in this paper indicate that its authors were not yet aware of the risk common to any neurogenic bladder, Pdet. In meningomyelocele patients, VUR is directly related to Pdet in that it is pressure-driven. Control of pressure is thus an essential element in the treatment of the neurogenic bladder in this patient population. Given that bacteriuria is almost always present and cannot be eradicated and that rigid control of Pdet ameliorates risk, one's attention should be directed at that variable and not at a primary effort to eradicate bacteriuria, which is not possible.

Perkash[25] noted that in contrast to those managed by sphincterotomy, patients with spinal injury managed by intermittent catheterization sometimes develop what he called "silent hydronephrosis." He meant that on routine imaging, seemingly stable patients had hydronephrosis. These patients were not monitored by urodynamic testing, which illustrates that without control of Pdet, intermittent catheterization is dangerous. The same can be said about sphincterotomy or any method of management of the neurogenic bladder that does not rely on control of bladder pressure. Until recently, the most common way to control bladder pressure and incontinence was an indwelling catheter, but that had its own serious and cumulative complications.

The identification of Pdet as a risk factor in neurogenic bladder dysfunction

Probably the first single paper on Pdet as a risk factor was published in 1978 by Light and coworkers,[26] describing upper tract deterioration in children with myelodysplasia. This paper was published in the South African Journal of Surgery and was not recognized as generally applicable to all neurogenic bladder conditions until later and certainly was not applied to the myelodysplastic population until much later. In 1981, McGuire and coworkers[27] reported that upper tract damage in a large group of myelodysplastic children was related to the Pdet required to induce leakage. Not all patients with high Pdet had upper tract deterioration at the time of the report, but all children with a high detrusor leak point pressure ultimately did develop upper tract disease when followed up by McGuire and colleagues[28] in 1983. Ghoneim and coworkers,[29] in 1989, studied a group of myelodysplastic children and found that those with higher leak point pressures had low-compliance bladders and an equally high rate of upper tract deterioration. Clinical outcomes vastly improved once that association was made, and treatment by intermittent catheterization was supplemented with drug therapy to control bladder pressure, or a procedure to decrease outlet resistance was initiated as directed by pressure monitoring. Subsequently, there have been multiple papers in the literature on Pdet as the risk factor in neurogenic vesical dysfunction. Baskin and coworkers[30] used anticholinergic agents and intermittent catheterization in myelodysplastic children with good success. Any improvement in the 39% to 48% upper tract damage rate recorded in these children before the recognition that Pdet was the problem was a huge step forward. The 39% upper tract deterioration rate is that recorded from the University of Michigan population in Ann Arbor, well after intermittent catheterization had been established as a method of treatment in these patients. The 48% number comes from another study in which children were observed but not treated with intermittent catheterization. The improvement in outcome was the result of bladder pressure management, not solely the result of clean intermittent catheterization and certainly not the result of antimicrobial therapy. Patients treated by drugs and clean intermittent catheterization were at least as bacteriuric as those patients not so treated and perhaps more so. Park and coworkers,[31] in 2001, reported on their institutional experience with sphincter dilation in myelodysplastic children monitored by the effect of that procedure on the detrusor leak point pressure and bladder compliance. The initial goal was a transient reduction in leak point pressure, buying time so that the child could avoid a cutaneous vesicostomy. An unexpected benefit was a dramatic and sustained effect on bladder compliance. This study duplicated the findings reported by Bloom and coworkers[32] in 1990 on sphincter dilation in myelodysplastic patients. These 2 studies and the effect of cutaneous vesicostomy on bladder compliance, upper tract integrity, and vesicoureteral reflux confirmed the role of the outlet in the genesis of the dangerous Pdet (Connolly and colleagues,[33] 1998). Elevated urethral resistance starts a process in which compliance deteriorates and Pdets increase. Ureteral work increases as a result but reaches a limit at about 40 cm of water ambient bladder pressure, whereupon ureteral delivery of urine to the bladder ceases. This is not due to the thickness of the bladder wall but rather, to transmission of Pdet to the ureter. However, ureteral dilation and the other effects on the ureter seen by radiography are late rather than immediate changes. For example, Ozkan and coworkers,[34] in 2005, studied a group of patients with severe bladder dysfunction that led to augmentation cystoplasty. They found an elevated detrusor leak point pressure and detrusor fibrosis, with poor storage behavior being the major risk factor for upper urinary tract deterioration. Ghoneim and coworkers[35] noted in a 1990 paper that outlet obstruction associated with detrusor leak point pressure greater than 40 cm was the most important risk factor in children with neurogenic vesical dysfunction and that early treatment predicated on urodynamic findings could prevent upper tract damage. Kaufman and colleagues,[36] in 1996, and Flood and colleagues,[37] in 1994, compared upper tract outcomes in myelodysplastic children monitored by periodic urodynamic testing with the outcome in myelodysplastic children followed by radiographic observation only. The urodynamic testing identified elevated detrusor leak point pressures and led to early treatment and prevention of upper tract damage. This was not the case in children followed by radiographic surveillance. Treatment in the radiographic group was instituted later and, in many cases, late enough so as not to prevent damage to upper tract function. Wang and coworkers[4] described a pressure management system for the neurogenic bladder in 1988, which was generally adapted with modifications by those caring for patients with neurogenic vesical dysfunction. For example, Kim and coworkers[38] reported in 1998 that they used bladder leak point pressure as the measure of success of sphincterotomy, rather than the more traditional measurement of residual urine. Perkash,[25] in 1978, suggested that voiding pressure did not always identify patients with detrusor sphincter dyssynergia who required a sphincterotomy.

That was in the early days of long-term clean intermittent catheterization, and some workers found sphincterotomy in male patients to be more effective long-term management than clean intermittent catheterization. Conversely, by the 1990s, it was clear that the effect of sphincterotomy was on Pdet; though effective, there were disadvantages to that technique, namely incontinence.

Failure of treatment of the neurogenic bladder

However improved the ability to predict upper tract changes based on urodynamic testing, there are cases in which damage has already been done or a treatment does not bring about a satisfactory reduction in bladder pressure. In such cases, continence is also a problem, along with the ongoing risk to upper tract function. For these situations, procedures to enlarge the bladder have been used successfully. Esa and coworkers,[39] in 1990, reported on 15 patients with low bladder compliance associated with various conditions that were treated by augmentation cystoplasty, with successful resolution of bladder dysfunction and incontinence and maintenance of normal upper urinary tracts. Blavais and coworkers,[40] in 2005, reported late outcomes after augmentation cystoplasty in a diverse group of patients. Mean bladder capacity increased from 166 to 522 mL and end Pdet, or Pdet at capacity, changed from 53 to 14. Flood and coworkers,[41] in 1995, reported on 122 augmentation cystoplasties done over a 10-year period. Bladder capacity increased from a mean of 108 mL to 448 mL and upper tract deterioration ceased after augmentation cystoplasty. Krishna and Gough,[42] in 1994, studied 39 children treated by augmentation cystoplasty for abnormal bladder compliance and vesicoureteral reflux. They noted that an achieved reduction in storage pressure below 20 was associated with cessation of vesicoureteral reflux without ureteral reimplantation. Even more telling are the reports of augmentation cystoplasty before renal transplantation in patients whose renal failure was the result of poor bladder function. Zaragoza and coworkers,[43] in 1993, reported excellent results with pretransplant augmentation cystoplasty in 11 patients in whom renal failure was caused by bladder dysfunction. In 2005, similar results were reported by Mendizabal and coworkers,[44] who reported on 15 patients with renal failure related to bladder dysfunction operated on between 1979 and 2003. Seven of 15 patients had an augmentation cystoplasty, others an ileal loop diversion or a vesicostomy. Graft survival rates after transplantation were similar to those in persons with normal bladder function. In 2002, Nahas and coworkers[45] reported on 21 patients with renal failure due to severe bladder dysfunction. All 21 patients had an augmentation cystoplasty, with excellent graft survival at 53 months.

Problems with augmentation cystoplasty

There is no question that augmentation cystoplasty is effective in the treatment of low-compliance or hyper-reflexic bladder. The procedure corrects vesicoureteral reflux, improves continence function, and protects the upper urinary tract, and late outcomes are excellent. On balance, the risks posed by a poorly compliant bladder justify the use of bowel segments for bladder enlargement if bladder compliance is not successfully treated by other means. There are still serious problems related to augmentation cystoplasty, including stone formation in as many as 30%; spontaneous perforation in 7% to 20%; progression of upper tract disease, which is rare; bowel obstruction and mucus production, both lifetime risks; nocturnal incontinence; electrolyte disturbance; vitamin deficiency; chronic infection; pyelonephritis; need for intermittent catheterization; and potential development of malignancy in the augmented bladder. Augmentation cystoplasties are generally effective reasonably quickly in the postoperative period. However, not all bladder augmentations are equally effective. To ensure the desired objective, reduction of Pdet to all volumes seen by the augmented bladder on a daily basis, patients who have an augmentation cystoplasty should be monitored frequently with urodynamic studies for the first year or two after the procedure. This can only be done urodynamically by a determination of the bladder pressure achieved by a given augmented bladder to the maximum volume recovered on intermittent catheterization.

Complications related directly to augmentation

Bertschy and coworkers,[46] in 2000, reported on complications of augmentation cystoplasty in children. In a cohort of 30 patients, 21 had recurrent symptomatic infections; 5, bladder stones; 3, intestinal volvulus; and 1, severe electrolyte disturbances. Rigaud and Le Normand,[47] in 2004, noted chronic bacteriuria in a high percentage of patients and a 10% to 15% incidence of stone formation. They estimated the rate of perforation to be 10% to 15%. In the large series consisting of 122 augmentation cystoplasty patients reported by Flood and coworkers[41] in 1995, 16% had a surgical revision of the augmentation, 21% developed bladder stones, and, of these, 30% had more than one episode of stone formation. Urinary incontinence occurred in 13% and required treatment in 6 patients and pyelonephritis was reported in 11%, but this is not very often documented by specific measures and tends to be recorded when these patients are seen by other practitioners, because they are always bacteriuric. Five patients developed a bowel obstruction and 4% had spontaneous perforation. Admittedly, this was a seriously ill population before augmentation cystoplasty, but these complications are nevertheless notable. In 2005, in a rigorous study of outcome after augmentation cystoplasty in 76 patients, Blavais and coworkers,[40] noted that although they achieved good bladder capacity and very low bladder pressures, 7 patients with interstitial cystitis failed to improve, 5 had chronic diarrhea, 11 of 26 with a stoma developed incontinence or stomal stenosis, and 4% developed renal or reservoir stones.

Malignancy is another serious problem in patients with a neurogenic bladder. Although there are definite concerns about malignant tumor development after augmentation cystoplasty, in 2003 at the West Roxbury VA Spinal Cord Injury Center, Hess and coworkers[48] noted that cancer of the bladder developed 16 to 28 times more frequently in patients with neurogenic bladder dysfunction than a normal age-matched population, even in the absence of augmentation cystoplasty. Therefore, other factors are involved in tumor development in these patients.

Nevertheless, there are numerous reports of the development of malignant tumors in the bladder remnant or bowel segment used for augmentation cystoplasty. Barrington and coworkers,[49] in 1997, reported 4 adenocarcinomas arising in the bladder remnant after augmentation cystoplasty. They concluded that these were urothelial in origin. Baydar,[50] in 2005, reported the development of a signet ring carcinoma in a gastrocystoplasty. There are reports of squamous cell carcinoma, adenocarcinoma, and transitional cell carcinoma developing in augmented bladders. They include reports from more than 10 centers. The exact rate of increase in the incidence of malignancy after augmentation cystoplasty is not clear. This lack of clarity can be attributed to (1) the risk of malignant transformation in neurogenic bladders in general and (2) the not unreasonable assumption that malignancy developing after bowel augmentation is more likely to be reported than that which develops when neurogenic bladder dysfunction is managed without augmentation. This is currently an unknown. What is known is that augmentation cystoplasty tends to be done in young and even very young people.

The incubation time for malignant transformation seems to be long, and there are no well-established methods of surveillance, although periodic endoscopy and cytology have been advocated. The sensitivity and specificity of these methods has not been established (Hamid and colleagues,[51] 2003).

Other methods to control bladder pressure

Several other treatments to decrease Pdet are in use. These include autoaugmentation, electrical stimulation, vibratory stimulation, and botulinum toxin injection into the detrusor muscle or the external sphincter. Autoaugmentation was described by Cartwright and Snow[52] in 1989 and has been used in some centers with good and not-so-good results. Stohrer and coworkers,[53] in 1999, reported good results in 62 patients with spinal cord lesions from the Spinal Cord Injury Center in Murnau, Germany. MacNeilly and coworkers,[54] in 2003, reported poor long-term outcomes after autoaugmentation in children with neuropathic dysfunction.

Botulinum toxin injected into the detrusor muscle or external sphincter is effective as reported by Schurch[55] and Schmidt and coworkers[56] in 2006. The effects are transient, lasting up to 7 months, and the material is expensive.

Sacral root stimulation combined with dorsal root section has been used for many years to control Pdet and autonomic dysreflexia and to stimulate voiding. In centers with experience, results are generally excellent. In 2003, Vastenholt and coworkers[57] reported a series of 42 patients with excellent results. There are numerous reports from Europe, Canada, and the United States with similar data; for example, Kutzenberger and colleagues[58] in 2005 reporting Deiter Sauerwein's extensive experience with some 440 cases over a 17-year period.

Vibratory stimulation intended to induce ejaculation in spinal cord-injured men had an unexpected side effect: modulation of detrusor activity that was quite profound. Laessoe and coworkers[59] reported on these effects in 2001 from Denmark. Clinical trials have started, and devices for this kind of stimulation are being tested.

To a large extent, these newer treatment methods were the result of dissatisfaction with certain aspects of augmentation cystoplasty enumerated earlier. However, all these treatments are designed to control bladder pressure, and evaluation of their efficacy is determined by urodynamic testing and in clinical outcome. Early on in the course of an injury or in the life of a child with myelodysplasia, adequate control of bladder pressure can be achieved with drugs and intermittent catheterization. It can also be achieved by reduction in outlet resistance, but that is also problematic. However, there is a link between outlet resistance and poor compliance. The effects of a reduction in outlet resistance are complex, and they are not described simply by a lower leak point pressure. In spinal cord injury patients with detrusor sphincter dyssynergia, myelodysplastic patients with elevated detrusor leak point pressures, and adult men with high-grade benign prostatic hyperplasia, there are definite and sustained improvements in bladder storage function and compliance that follow a reduction in outlet resistance. Because altered compliance is the major risk factor for upper tract damage and incontinence, this is the desired outcome. A reduction in outlet resistance cannot be said to be superior to intermittent catheterization, because the latter favors preservation of continence. There are still cases in which bladder function cannot be improved by medication, clean intermittent catheterization, and the other measures mentioned earlier, possibly because the process is so long-standing that the bladder muscles have been replaced by fibrous tissue. In these cases, bladder enlargement procedures still have value. Augmentation cystoplasty has definitely altered the natural history of neurogenic vesical dysfunction, in that it reliably controls bladder pressure. Should patients be selected by urodynamic testing for early intensive intervention, the rate of augmentation cystoplasty would probably be dramatically decreased.

Urodynamics and the neurogenic bladder

The goal of any therapy for the neurogenic bladder is to keep Pdets within very narrow limits, thus preserving upper tract integrity and continence. There are a few rules. Compliance on the bladder pressure response in incremental volume is the most important single test of risk. Compliance can be measured by a simple cystometrogram or more complex urodynamics, including the subtracted pressure system in which abdominal pressure measured with a rectal catheter is continuously subtracted from bladder pressure to provide true Pdet. This can be supplemented with an electromyographic recording of the activity of the external sphincter and video observation of the bladder, urethra, and ureters during the study to provide more information. However, for measured compliance to be meaningful, it must be determined over the volume range actually seen by the bladder studied. For example, a 33–year-old man with a T6 spinal cord injury is treated with 3 medications to control Pdet and provide continence. He catheterizes himself every 4 to 6 hours and obtains, as a maximum volume, 560 mL. He has never achieved a volume higher than 600 mL. His urodynamic testing must determine that his bladder compliance is acceptable for the entire volume range his bladder sees on a daily basis: 1 to 600 mL. Safe bladder pressures are less than 20 at all volumes. Somewhat higher pressures at terminal volumes in a given bladder are not harmful, but as a general rule, one aims for a Pdet less than 20. In another example, a 39-year-old man with multiple sclerosis is not capable of self-catheterization. He has, on initial urodynamic testing, a residual urine of 549 mL, and at 800 mL, he has a sustained high pressure detrusor contraction with detrusor sphincter dyssynergia. A Pdet of 122 cm is recorded over a 40-second time period with little or no flow. Obviously, bladder compliance in this patient from 0 to 549 mL is not important. This bladder only sees volumes from 549 to 800+ mL. Whatever the treatment, medication and clean intermittent catheterization, sphincterotomy and condom catheter drainage, or (as we chose) Botox A 100 units injected into the external sphincter, precise data on bladder capacity and mean residual urine volume is required to accurately evaluate bladder compliance.

In this case, at 1 month post-Botox, postvoid residual volume was 132 and a voiding contraction occurred at 500 mL. Compliance was slightly abnormal from 300 to capacity, but Pdet was less than 20 and voiding pressure at mid flow was 34. This is an acceptable result.

As a rule, in patients with neurogenic bladders who report stable urinary tract function, either a compliance test or an upper tract study should be done on a yearly basis. Of these, urodynamic testing is more accurate and provides much better prognostic data.

For those patients who report a febrile or symptomatic UTI, it is imperative that a compliance study and an upper tract evaluation be done quickly. Treatment of a UTI does not solve the problem in most patients with neurogenic bladder dysfunction, and the infection only recurs unless the functional problem is identified. In most cases, the problem involves bladder pressure.

Patients who report incontinence should also be studied, because in most cases, incontinence is the result of uncontrolled bladder pressure. Most of these patients would have been treated for the incontinence with antibiotics before the urologist knows about them, so forget that as a cause. It rarely is the sole cause of any problem in this population.

Spinal cord injury

After recovery from spinal shock, a period of quite rapid evolution of bladder and urethral function occurs. Bladders progress from low-pressure compliant systems to high-pressure obstructed systems quite quickly. Regular periodic urodynamic testing is essential. Caught early, the bladder responses to volume can be controlled with medication. Once high pressures are well established, it is more difficult to reverse them and recreate a low-pressure environment. Given a chance, medication is started before reflex bladder contractility is established in the hope of preventing it entirely. Rarely, if the spinal cord injury is partial and incomplete and recovery occurs, the drugs can be stopped without harm. After 18 months to 2 years, stable bladder dysfunction is usually achieved but cannot be assumed. Moreover, bladder function continues to slowly evolve and should still be monitored.

Sphincterotomy patients

Periodic evaluation, especially in patients with cervical lesions, is mandatory on a 6-month to 1-year basis, by testing the Pdet at which urine flows from the external meatus and not by a measurement of residual urine. This is a detrusor leak point pressure, the pressure at which flow past the distal sphincter occurs, and it requires fluoroscopy, but if that is not available, watching for urine to egress from the external meatus is acceptable. If the pressure is 5 or less, all is well. If it is higher, caution and frequent testing are required. The sphincterotomy should be redone if pressures climb toward 30 or 35. A small urodynamic catheter is ideal for this and all other testing described in this article.

The International Continence Society's definition of a detrusor leak point pressure is the lowest pressure in the absence of a detrusor contraction or a change in abdominal pressure (Pabd) causing urine flow—a good definition, but wrong, because in that case, there would be no flow. The detrusor leak point pressure is the Pdet at which there is urine flow past the distal sphincter. The Pdet can be a result of a phasic contraction, poor compliance, and/or fibrosis of the bladder, but the measurement is of Pdet, however produced. That definition specifically excludes Pabd as the expulsive force.

NEOBLADDER AND AUGMENTATION CYSTOPLASTY PATIENTS

These patients take time to develop capacity, and any unexplained incontinence or febrile UTI should be promptly evaluated. These are complex situations and video testing is best, because bilateral high-grade VUR may occur, which renders compliance testing useless. Where reservoir pressures are elevated, medical therapy can be used, guided by repeat urodynamics. If there is leakage from a neourethra, the cause can be determined with video urodynamics. Leakage at low reservior pressure is likely the result of a dysfunctional flap valve, whereas leakage at high reservior storage pressure is more likely related to impaired reservoir compliance.

REFERENCES

1. Bors E, Comarr AE. Neurological urology. Baltimore (MD): University Park Press; 1971.
2. Devivo MJ, Black KJ, Stover SL. Causes of death during the first 12 years after spinal cord injury. Arch Phys Med Rehabil 1993;74:248.
3. Kasabian NG, Bauer SB, Dyro FM, et al. The prophylactic value of clean intermittent catheterization and anticholinergic medication in newborns and infants risk of developing urinary tract deterioration. Am J Dis Child 1992;146:840.
4. Wang SC, McGuire EJ, Bloom DA. A bladder pressure management system for myelodysplasia – clinical outcome. J Urol 1988;140:1499.
5. Cass AS, Giest RW. Results of conservative and surgical management of the neurogenic bladder in 160 children. J Urol 1972;107:865.
6. Bauer SB, Colodny AH, Retik AB. The management of vesicoureteral reflux in children with myelodysplasia. J Urol 1982;128:102.
7. Sidi AA, Peng W, Gonzalez R. Vesicoureteral refllux in children with myelodysplasia: natural history and results of treatment. J Urol 1986;136:329.

8. Simforoosh N, Tabibi A, Basiri A, et al. Is ureteral reimplantation necessary during augmentation cystoplasty in patients with neurogenic bladder and vesicoureteral reflux. J Urol 2002;168:1439.
9. Momose H, Okajima E, Yasukawa M, et al. [Unresolved issues concerning the operative indication of augmentation cystoplasty in spina bifida patients: a report of two patients]. Hinyokika Kiyo 1993;39: 747 [in Japanese].
10. Shapiro SR, Lebowitz R, Colodny AH. Fate of 90 children with ileal conduit urinary diversion a decade after: analysis of complications, pyelography, renal function and bacteriology. J Urol 1975;114:289.
11. Cass AS, Lunenberg M, Gleich P, et al. A 22-year follow-up of ileal conduits in children with a neurogenic bladder. J Urol 1984;132:529.
12. Mitchell ME, Yoder IC, Pfister RC, et al. Ileal loop stenosis: a late complication of urinary diversion. J Urol 1975;118:957.
13. Simeone C, Antonelli A, Tonini C, et al. Ileal conduit and urinary stoma complications. Arch Ital Urol Androl 2003;75:6–9.
14. Pastor DM, Pauli EM, Koltan WA, et al. Parastomal hernia repair: a single center experience. JSLS 2009;13:170–5.
15. Wan J, Fleenor S, Kielczewski P, et al. Urinary tract status of patients with neurogenic dysfunction presenting with upper tract stone disease. J Urol 1992;148:1126.
16. Breza J, Alemayehu HM, Hornak M, et al. Advantages of converting incontinent to continent urinary diversion. Int Urol Nephrol 1994;26:447.
17. Hetet JF, Rigaud J, Karam G, et al. Complications of Bricker ileal conduit urinary diversion: analysis of a series of 246 patients. Prog Urol 2005;15:23 [in French].
18. Whitmore WF, Fam BA, Yalla SV. Experience with anteromedian external sphincterotomy in 100 male subjects with neuropathic bladders. Br J Urol 1978;50:99.
19. Petri E, Waltz PH, Jonas U. Transurethral bladder neck operation in neurogenic bladder. Eur Urol 1978;4:189.
20. Lapides J, Diokno AC, Silber SJ, et al. Clean intermittent self catheterization in the treatment of urinary tract disease. J Urol 2000;167:1131.
21. Lapides J. Mechanisms of urinary tract infection. Urology 1979;14:217.
22. Last PM, Harbison PA, Marsh JA. Bacteraemia after urological instrumentation. Lancet 1966;1 (7428):74.
23. Barton CH, Vaziri ND, Gordon S, et al. Renal pathology in end stage renal disease associated with paraplegia. Paraplegia 1984;22:31.
24. Kass EJ, Koff SA, Diokno AC, et al. The significance of bacilluria in children on long term intermittent catheterization. J Urol 1981;126:223.
25. Perkash I. Detrusor sphincter dyssynergia and dyssynergic responses: recognition and rationale for early modified transurethral sphincterotomy in complete spinal cord injury lesions. J Urol 1978;120:469.
26. Light K, Cinman A, Giles GR, et al. Urodynamics in congenital neuropathic bladder. S Afr J Surg 1978; 16:237.
27. McGuire EJ, Woodside JR, Borden TA, et al. Prognostic value of urodynamic testing in myelodysplastic patients. J Urol 2002;167:1049 (reprint from a classic article from J Urol 1981).
28. McGuire EJ, Woodside JR, Borden TA. Upper tract deterioration in patients with myelodysplasia and detrusor hypertonia: a follow up study. J Urol 1983; 129:823.
29. Ghoneim GM, Bloom DA, McGuire EF, et al. Bladder compliance in meningomyelocele children. J Urol 1989;141:1404.
30. Baskin LS, Kogan BA, Benard F. Treatment of infants with neurogenic bladder dysfunction using anticholinergic drugs and intermittent catheterization. Br J Urol 1990;66:532.
31. Park JM, McGuire EJ, Koo HP, et al. External urethral sphincter dilation for the management of high risk meningomyelocele: 15 year experience. J Urol 2001;165:2838.
32. Bloom DA, Knechtel JM, McGuire EJ. Urethral dilation improves bladder compliance in children with myelomeningocele and high leak point pressure. J Urol 1990;144:430.
33. Conolly B, Fitzgerald RJ, Guiney EJ. Has vesicostomy a role in the neuropathic bladder. Z Kinderchir 1988;43(Suppl 2):17.
34. Ozkan B, Demirkesen O, Durak H, et al. Which factors predict upper urinary tract deterioration in overactive neurogenic bladder dysfunction. Urology 2005;66:99.
35. Ghoneim GM, Roach MB, Lewis VH, et al. The value of leak point pressure and bladder compliance in the urodynamic evaluation of myelomeningocele patients. J Urol 1990;144:1440.
36. Kaufman AM, Ritchey ML, Roberts AC, et al. Decreased bladder compliance in patients with myelomeningocele treated with radiological observation. J Urol 1996;156:2031.
37. Flood HD, Ritchey ML, Bloom DA, et al. Outcome of reflux in children with myelodysplasia managed by bladder pressure monitoring. J Urol 1994;152: 1574.
38. Kim YH, Kattan MW, Boone TB. Bladder leak point pressure: the measure for sphincterotomy success in spinal cord injured patients with external detrusor-sphincter dyssynergia. J Urol 1998;159:493.
39. Esa A, Uchida A, Kiwamoto H, et al. [Review of 14 year experience of augmentation enterocystoplasty. Observations on bowel dynamics]. Nippon Hinyokika Gakkai Zasshi 1990;81:713 [in Japanese].

40. Blavais JG, Weiss JP, Desai P, et al. Long-term follow-up of augmentation enterocystoplasty and continent diversion in patients with benign disease. J Urol 2005;173:1631.
41. Flood HD, Malhotra SJ, O'Connell HE, et al. Long-term results and complications using augmentation cystoplasty in reconstructive urology. Neurourol Urodyn 1995;14:297.
42. Krishna A, Gough DC. Evaluation of augmentation cystoplasty in childhood with reference to vesicoureteral reflux and urinary infection. Br J Urol 1994;74:465.
43. Zaragoza MR, Ritchey ML, Bloom DA, et al. Enterocystoplasty in renal transplantation candidates: urodynamic evaluation and outcome. J Urol 1993; 150:1463.
44. Mendizabal S, Estornell F, Zamora I, et al. Renal transplantation in children with severe bladder dysfunction. J Urol 2005;173:226.
45. Nahas WC, Mazzucchi E, Arap MA, et al. Augmentation cystoplasty in renal Transplantation a good and safe option. Experience with 25 cases. Urology 2002;60:770.
46. Bertschy C, Bawab F, Valioulis I, et al. Enterocystoplasty complications in children. A study of thirty cases. Eur J Pediatr Surg 2000;10:30.
47. Rigaud J, LeNormand L. Augmentation cystoplasty. Ann Urol (Paris) 2004;38:298.
48. Hess MJ, Zahn EH, Foo DK, et al. Bladder cancer in patients with spinal cord injury. J Spinal Cord Med 2003;26:322.
49. Barrington JW, Fulford S, Griffiths D, et al. Tumors in bladder after enterocystoplasty. J Urol 1997;157:485.
50. Baydar DE, Allan RW, Castellan M, et al. Anaplastic signet ring cell carcinoma arising in gastrocystoplasty. Urology 2005;65:1226.
51. Hamid R, Bycroft J, Arya M, et al. Screening cystoscopy and biopsy in patients with neuropathic bladder and chronic suprapubic indwelling catheters: is it valid. J Urol 2004;171:810 [A letter commenting on these methods of screening in spinal cord injury patients in response to a paper which used them. See J Urol 2003;170:425].
52. Cartwright PC, Snow BW. Bladder auto augmentation: early clinical experience. J Urol 1989;142:505.
53. Stohrer M, Goepel M, Kramer G, et al. [Detrusor myectomy in the treatment of hyper- reflexive low compliance bladder]. Urologe A 1999;38:30 [in German].
54. MacNeilly AE, Afshar K, Coleman GU, et al. Auto augmentation by detrusor myotomy: its lack of effectiveness in the management of congenital neuropathic bladder. J Urol 2003;170:1643.
55. Schurch B. Botulinum toxin for the management of bladder dysfunction. Drugs 2006;66:1301.
56. Schmidt DM, Sauermann P, Schuessler B, et al. Experience with 100 cases treated With Botulinum – A Toxin in the detrusor muscle for idiopathic overactive bladder syndrome refractory to anticholinergics. J Urol 2006;176:177.
57. Vastenholt JM, Snoek GJ, Buschman HP, et al. A 7-year follow-up of sacral anterior root stimulation for bladder control in patients with spinal cord injury: quality of life and users' experience. Spinal Cord 2003;41:397.
58. Kutzenberger J, Domurath B, Sauerwein D. Spastic bladder and spinal cord injury: 17 years of experience with sacral differentiation and implantation of an anterior root stimulator. Artif Organs 2005;29:239.
59. Laessoe L, Sonksen J, Bagi P, et al. Effects of ejaculation by penile vibratory stimulation of bladder capacity in men with spinal cord lesions. J Urol 2003;169:2216.

Review of Neurologic Diseases for the Urologist

Clare J. Fowler, FRCP*, Catherine Dalton, MRCPI,
Jalesh N. Panicker, MD, DM, MRCP (UK)

KEYWORDS

- Neurology of bladder control • Frontal lobes
- Geriatric incontinence • MSA • Parkinson's disease
- Multiple sclerosis

Many different neurologic pathologies can affect the central and peripheral nervous system resulting in neurogenic incontinence. A list of these is given in **Box 1** and in depth discussion of these conditions can be found in standard text books.[1,2] However, this article attempts to update the urologist on recent developments that have altered the neurologic understanding of a select group of diseases that have a particularly high incidence of bladder dysfunction.

FRONTAL LOBE FUNCTION AND DISEASE

Although frontal lobe lesions have been known to produce bladder function disturbances since the publication of Andrew and Nathan[3] in 1964, recent findings based on functional brain imaging techniques have greatly enhanced understanding and knowledge of the importance of this brain region for bladder control. Based on an analysis of both the positron emission tomography (PET) and functional MRI (fMRI) studies, a working model of lower urinary tract control by higher brain centers was proposed in a recent review article,[4] an illustration from which is shown in **Fig. 1**.

As anticipated from the results of animal experimental studies, the primary relay center for bladder afferents is now known to be a midbrain structure, the periaqueductal gray (PAG). This region has rich connections with pelvic organs, and it has been proposed that it has an important role in homeostasis and reproductive function.[5] Activation of the PAG has now been shown in many studies of the effect of bladder filling, as illustrated by a recent meta-analysis of the literature by Griffiths and Tadic **Fig. 2**.[6]

The pontine micturition center (PMC) (see **Figs. 1** and **2**), formerly known as *Barrington's nucleus*, is the brainstem region that connects directly to the sacral spinal cord, and its activation effects relaxation of the striated urethral sphincter followed by contraction of the detrusor muscle. The existence of an additional brain stem region, the L-region (see **Fig. 2**), activated during withholding micturition, is less clear.[6] Current theory maintains that the PMC in humans does not receive direct bladder afferent input, but rather is "informed" by the PAG. The PMC is held in a state of inhibition by the PAG throughout bladder filling while continence is maintained through social considerations.[7] Consciousness about the appropriateness of voiding is provided by input from higher centers, specifically the medial prefrontal cortex and the hypothalamus, with this input modulating PAG activity.

While inhibiting micturition, higher cerebral regions are also activated by bladder filling, and the right insula is particularly recognized as being

This work was undertaken at the University College London Hospitals/University College London, which received a proportion of funding from the Department of Health's NIHR Biomedical Research Centres funding scheme.
UCL Institute of Neurology and National Hospital for Neurology and Neurosurgery, UCLH, Box 71, Queen Square, London WC1N 3BG, UK
* Corresponding author.
E-mail address: c.fowler@ion.ucl.ac.uk

Urol Clin N Am 37 (2010) 517–526
doi:10.1016/j.ucl.2010.07.004
0094-0143/10/$ – see front matter

urologic.theclinics.com

Box 1
Neurologic disorders causing lower urinary tract dysfunction

Suprapontine causes
Stroke
Traumatic brain injury
Degeneration
Parkinson's disease
multiple system atrophy
Alzheimer's disease
Hydrocephalus, normal pressure hydrocephalus
Cerebral palsy
Neoplasm
Infrapontine-suprasacral causes
Demyelination
Multiple sclerosis
Transverse myelitis
Trauma
Vascular
Arteriovenous malformations
Spinal cord infarction
Neoplasm
Metastasis
Primary
Hereditary
Hereditary spastic paraparesis
Infections
Tropical spastic paraparesis (HTLV-I)
Spina bifida
Infrasacral causes
Cauda equina damage
Diabetes mellitus
Hereditary
Hereditary motor sensory neuropathy
Pelvic surgery

an important structure in the process of "interoception." Interoception can be defined as "the sense of the physiologic condition of the entire body," and recently Craig[8] emphasized that this includes the sensations of pain and temperature and visceral sensations. From the insula, activity is processed in the lateral prefrontal cortex and therefore acquires "hedonic valency," or a qualitative value as to pleasantness or otherwise. The anterior cingulate cortex (ACC) is part of the limbic system, a network of brain regions involved in the processing and generation of emotions. The ACC is now thought to have an important role as the efferent system for autonomic activity.

AGING AND INCONTINENCE

Symptoms of an overactive bladder and urgency incontinence have been shown to have an increasing prevalence with aging by many different studies, such as SIFO in Europe[9] and NOBLE in the United States.[10] Why this should be and what is the cause of the high incidence of incontinence in the elderly has long been uncertain. Although incontinence has long been known to be multifactorial, observational studies had shown that the disorder in the frail elderly was often associated with a degree of cognitive and functional decline and a tendency to falls, and therefore several risk factors seemed to be associated with incontinence, many unrelated to the genitourinary tract.[11] However, recent advances in this area have shown that white matter lesions, formerly considered an incidental finding on MRI and of little clinical relevance, are not as benign as previously thought,[12] but may instead be a significant factor in causing disconnections in brain areas critical to bladder control, such as those shown in **Fig. 1**. White matter hyperintensities (WMH) causing *leukoaraiosis*, or white matter wasting, are commonly present on the MRI scans of older people and have been linked to vascular risk factors.

The association between WMH and urinary incontinence in the elderly was first recognized by Sakakibara and Hattori[13] 1999. This Japanese group observed that although detrusor overactivity was found in 82% of elderly subjects with these MRI changes, it occurred in only 9% of those without. Furthermore, in those with mild leukoaraiosis, urinary incontinence was more common than was cognitive impairment or gait slowness, suggesting that urinary dysfunction is a common and early sign in elderly people with leukoaraiosis or white matter disease. These observations were subsequently confirmed[12,14] and the hypothesis developed that the white matter damage involves focal tracts connecting centers involved in bladder control (see **Fig. 1**). Using computer-based imaging techniques, both to identify connecting white matter tracts ands quantify the amount of white matter disease, the severity and degree of bother from incontinence was shown to be associated with a high burden of WMH in the right inferior frontal region and specific white matter tracts that connect frontal regions to other brain regions involved in maintaining continence.[15]

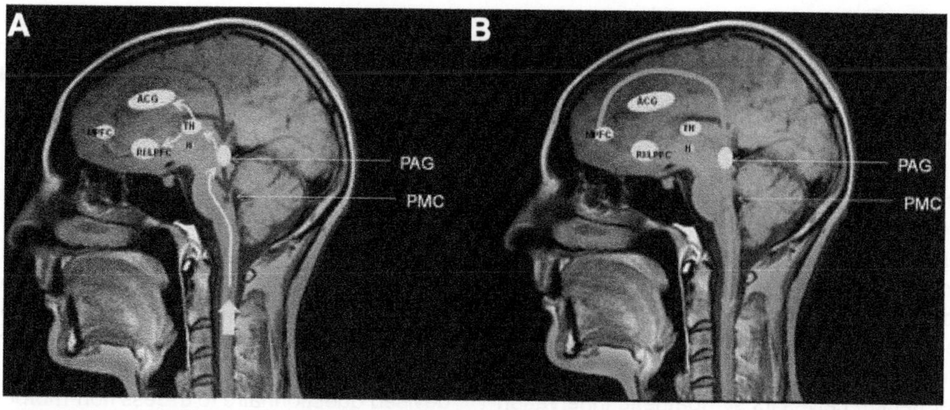

Fig. 1. A preliminary working model of lower urinary tract control by higher brain centers. (*A*) During storage, ascending afferents synapse on the midbrain periaqueductal gray (PAG); they are relayed via the hypothalamus (H) and thalamus (TH) to the dorsal anterior cingulate cortex (ACC), the right insula (RI), and the lateral prefrontal cortex (LPFC); in the storage phase they pass to the medial prefrontal cortex (MPFC), where the decision to void or not is made. During storage, the decision is not to void, and the condition is maintained through chronic inhibition of the PAG via a long pathway from the MPFC. Consequently, the pontine micturition center (PMC) is also suppressed, and voiding does not occur. (*B*) When the decision to void is made, the MPFC relaxes its inhibition of the PAG (*arrow*) and the hypothalamus (H) also provides a "safe" signal. Consequently, the PAG excites the PMC, which then sends descending motor output (*arrow*) to the sacral spinal cord, which ultimately relaxes the urethral sphincter and contracts the detrusor so that voiding occurs. Voiding is continued to completion through continuing afferent input, probably to the PAG. (*Reprinted from* Fowler, CJ, Griffiths DJ. A decade of functional brain imaging applied to bladder control. Neurourol Urodyn 2010;29(1):49–55; with permission.)

BLADDER SYMPTOMS IN MOVEMENT DISORDERS

Multiple System Atrophy

Multiple system atrophy (MSA) can present either as a poorly levodopa-responsive parkinsonism (MSA-P) or a cerebellar dysfunction (MSA-C), but in either condition, additional bladder dysfunction causing urinary incontinence is an early feature.[16]

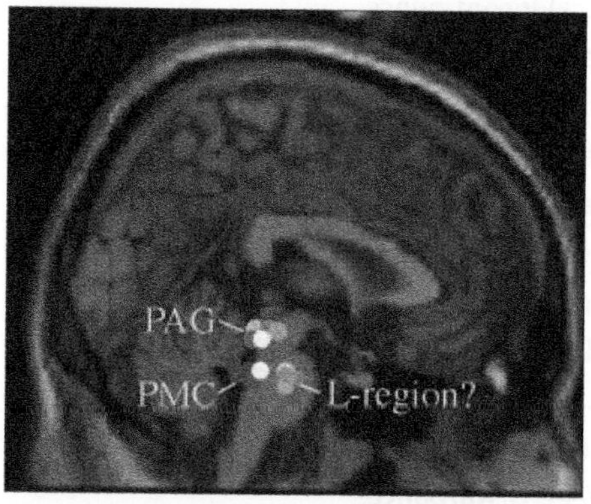

Fig. 2. Reported locations of peak activation (deactivation in a few cases) of brainstem areas activated during withholding of urine or full bladder, or during voiding, projected on a medial section of the brain (based on PET, fMRI, and single photon emission CT studies in healthy controls). (*Reprinted from* Griffiths D, Tadic SD. Bladder control, urgency, and urge incontinence: evidence from functional brain imaging. Neurourol Urodyn 2008;27(6):466–74; with permission.)

The differential diagnosis between MSA-P and the more common disease, Parkinson's disease, can be difficult even for neurologists who specialize in movement disorders. However, early troublesome incontinence and even earlier erectile dysfunction in men are now regarded as sinister warning signs that the neurologic condition may be the more rapidly fatal condition of MSA.[16] Frequency occurring during the day and night, urinary urgency, urgency incontinence, incomplete bladder emptying, urinary retention, or a combination of these disorders can occur, with the expected adverse effect on quality of life.[17]

Urodynamic investigations in patients with MSA commonly show detrusor overactivity as the underlying cause of overactive bladder symptoms.[18] Detrusor overactivity is thought to result from the central pathology of MSA, which includes neuronal loss of neuromelanin-containing cells in the nigrostriatal dopaminergic system, cerebellum, pontomedullary raphe (resulting in the MRI appearance of the pontine cross sign), and frontal cortex.[19,20]

Incomplete bladder emptying worsens with progression of the illness. A study measuring the postvoid residual volume in patients with MSA found a steady increase in mean postvoid residual between the first and fifth years.[21] Incomplete bladder emptying is now recognized as being so characteristic of the bladder disorder in MSA that the finding of a raised postvoid residual volume has been suggested as a useful discriminator in the differential diagnosis of MSA and Parkinson's disease.[22] The neurologic basis for this finding has yet to be fully elucidated, but it may be related to the MSA disease process affecting the descending spinal pathways to the sacral parasympathetic outflow.

The combination of detrusor overactivity and incomplete bladder emptying contribute to the prominent urinary incontinence characterizing this condition. Continence is further compromised by the development of an open bladder neck and weakness of the striated urethral sphincter. The bladder neck receives its sympathetic innervation from the hypogastric nerve, and the pathology of MSA commonly affects the interomedial lateral cell columns in the thoracic cord that convey descending sympathetic innervation, resulting in deficits that underlie the postural hypotension and the open bladder neck found in this condition.[23] In one study, an open bladder neck at the start of bladder filling without the accompanying bladder overactivity was found in 53% of patients with MSA but not in any with Parkinson's disease ($P<.01$).[18] An open bladder neck may be asymptomatic in women but, in combination with the other disorders of bladder function seen in MSA, contributes to incontinence.

Denervation of the striated sphincters is an abnormality that is fairly specific for MSA, resulting from loss of anterior horn cells in the Onuf's nucleus of the sacral spinal cord. This group of cells, first described by Onufrowicz in 1900, projects to the external sphincters and was found to show a selective loss in postmortem studies of patients dying with MSA. The striated urethral sphincter is critical for the maintenance of continence, and sphincter weakness in MSA may result in continuous urinary incontinence in female patients[24] and contribute to poor bladder control in both sexes.

As the anterior horn cells of Onuf's nuclei are spared in Parkinson's disease,[25] sphincter electromyogram (EMG) was proposed as a valuable means for distinguishing MSA-P from Parkinson's disease,[26,27] although others have not found the technique valuable.[28] The value of sphincter EMG as a test to distinguish MSA from Parkinson's disease has been greatly debated, but in a patient with a history of a cerebellar or akinetic rigid syndrome of less than 5 years and with significant urinary symptoms, a normal result makes the diagnosis of MSA unlikely.[29]

Parkinson's Disease

In recent years there has been increasing recognition that Parkinson's disease involves many brain regions other than the substantia nigra and that many of the non-motor symptoms of the condition reflect this multisystem involvement. Although many different agents are effective for treating the motor manifestations of this condition, such as levodopa and dopamine agonists, these do little to ameliorate the non-motor symptoms, such as those listed in **Box 2**.

Symptoms relating to pelvic organ dysfunctions rate highly among complaints that have an adverse effect on quality of life, with problems relating to the bladder particularly common. Recently an international survey used a newly devised questionnaire to assess non-motor symptoms of Parkinson's disease (NMSQuest) in a multinational survey of 545 patients with a mild disability.[30] Results reflected that 56% answered positively to the question "have you experienced a sense of urgency to pass urine which makes you rush to the toilet." However, the most common

Box 2
Non-motor symptoms in Parkinson's disease

Bladder disturbances

Nocturia

Urgency

Incontinence

Gastrointestinal disturbances

Dysphagia

Vomiting

Constipation

Fecal incontinence

Sexual Dysfunction

Erectile dysfunction

Reduced libido

Behavioral and cognitive changes

Depression

Anxiety

Memory loss

Poor concentration

Delusions

Sleep Disturbances

Hypersomnia

Insomnia

Vivid dreams

Rapid eye movement behavior disorder (enacting dreams)

Restless leg syndrome

of all complaints was nocturia, with 62% answering in the affirmative to the question "have you experienced getting up regularly at night to pass urine." That study showed that urinary-related questions had the highest percentage positive answers of all nine domains.[31] An earlier questionnaire study from Japan focusing only on pelvic organ symptoms, given to 115 patients with Parkinson's disease with only slightly worse disability than patients in the multinational study, found that 42% of women and 54% of men complained of urinary urgency, and that this incidence was significantly higher than an age-matched control group.[32]

Dopamine has an indirect inhibitory effect on the micturition reflex,[33,34] and detrusor overactivity in Parkinson's disease may result from a loss of inhibition of the reflex. Patients may also develop nocturnal polyuria in the course of the disease. The exact mechanism for this is unknown, although the circadian pattern of arginine-vasopressin release has been reported to be lost in experimental parkinsonism.[35]

Although less common than storage symptoms, voiding symptoms also occur in Parkinson's disease. Patients most commonly report hesitancy, straining to void, and a poor urinary stream; however, postvoid residuals are typically low.[32] Patients have been shown to have a weak detrusor during pressure flow studies,[18] and this may correlate with the stage of the disease.[36] Previous descriptions of pseudo-dyssynergia were attributed to Parkinson's disease through analogy with limb bradykinesia[37]; however, urodynamics has shown mild urethral obstruction.[18] The possibility that high resting urethral pressure may result from medications, levodopa, and its metabolites, such as norepinephrine, has been suggested.[38]

Neuropathologic studies now suggest that the pathology that affects the brain in Parkinson's disease—the disposition of Lewy bodies—starts in the dorsal motor nucleus of the vagus in the brain stem and in the olfactory bulb and tract. Parkinson's disease can be neuropathologically staged according to the ascending progression of Lewy bodies, only involving the substantia nigra at stage three of a total of six stages (**Fig. 3**). Phases one through three and may predate the onset of motor symptoms by many years, and according to this system, constipation is a feature of the presymptomatic phase.[39] However, the connection may be even more significant, and experts have hypothesized that an unidentified toxin passes through the mucosal barrier of the intestine and is transported in a retrograde manner by the vagus nerve axon, leading to vagal nucleus damage.[40]

The staging of the neuropathology of Parkinson's disease (see **Fig. 3**) serves as a valuable framework for understanding how the bladder symptoms occur in the context of a patient with Parkinson's disease with more severe disability than simply motor symptoms. The weight of evidence suggests that a correlation exists between the severity of neurologic disability and the occurrence of bladder symptoms in

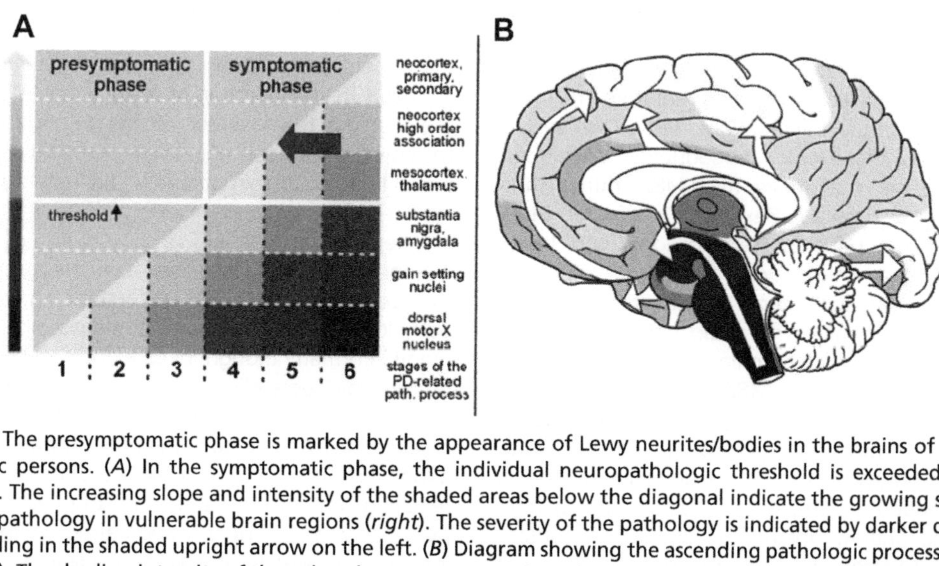

Fig. 3. The presymptomatic phase is marked by the appearance of Lewy neurites/bodies in the brains of asymptomatic persons. (*A*) In the symptomatic phase, the individual neuropathologic threshold is exceeded (*black arrow*). The increasing slope and intensity of the shaded areas below the diagonal indicate the growing severity of the pathology in vulnerable brain regions (*right*). The severity of the pathology is indicated by darker degrees of shading in the shaded upright arrow on the left. (*B*) Diagram showing the ascending pathologic process (*white arrows*). The shading intensity of the colored areas corresponds to that in *A*. The large arrow pointing just above stage 4 indicates the stage at which bladder symptoms become common. (*From* Braak H, Ghebremedhin E, Rub U, et al. Stages in the development of Parkinson's disease-related pathology. Cell Tissue Res 2004;318:121; with permission.)

Parkinson's disease, and therefore it seems reasonable to put the clinical threshold for bladder symptomatology above Braak stage four (ie, a point at which the neuropathology is starting to affect the neocortex; see large arrow **Fig. 3**). This theory explains why typically patients with Parkinson's disease in whom the bladder symptoms are from the neurologic disease (rather than prostatic symptoms; see later discussion) often show features that are particularly challenging to treat.

In contrast to constipation and disorders of the bowel, bladder dysfunction as part of Parkinson's disease occurs relatively late and is thought to result from central rather than peripheral nervous system abnormalities. Not all patients with Parkinson's disease develop bladder symptoms, although bladder symptoms are more predictably troublesome as the disease advances. A lack of correlation between the severity of neurological deficit in the early stages and onset of bladder symptoms in Parkinson's disease means that there may be considerable diagnostic difficulties, particularly in men with mild Parkinson's disease and lower urinary tract symptoms (LUTS). The symptoms of benign prostatic outflow include voiding difficulty, frequency and urgency and night-time frequency are symptoms that are particularly likely to be troublesome symptoms in the later stages of Parkinson's disease.

A highly influential paper describing the onset of urinary incontinence after prostatic surgery in patients with parkinsonism and poor voluntary sphincter contractions[41] seemed to make urologists very cautious about operating on men with Parkinson's disease. However, with the recognition which followed publication of that paper of the clinical features of MSA and the early incontinence in the disease, in retrospect it seems likely that some of the patients included in the series, particularly those who subsequently developed incontinence, may have had MSA rather than Parkinson's disease. Based on sphincter EMG findings, the patients were divided into those who could and those who could not voluntarily contract their sphincters, and it was observed that many of those who could not had changes of denervation and chronic reinnervation, as is now known to occur in MSA.

Experts now generally agree that the incontinence of MSA rarely improves after prostate surgery; however, men with a definitive diagnosis of Parkinson's disease and coincidental benign prostatic outflow obstruction should be considered for appropriate surgery. The incidence of incontinence in men undergoing radical prostatectomy for prostate cancer was the same for those with and without Parkinson's disease, and a recent retrospective study of 23 men with benign prostatic outflow obstruction who underwent a transurethral resection of the prostate (TURP) showed a 70% favorable response rate, the authors concluding that "in case of refractory voiding symptoms, the risk of de novo urinary incontinence seems minimal. Thus, TURP should not be considered contraindicated in patients with Parkinson's disease provided that preoperative investigations including urodynamic assessment indicate prostatic bladder outlet obstruction."[42]

Multiple Sclerosis: Progress With Treatment

In developed countries, multiple sclerosis is the most common neurologic disease that causes progressive neurologic disability in young people. The disease has several different subtypes: relapsing remitting, primary progressive, progressive relapsing, secondary progressive, or benign. The advent of MRI scanning changed the investigations needed to secure a diagnosis of multiple sclerosis. In a new case of multiple sclerosis, multiple periventricular lesions can be seen, which enhance with gadolinium when they first appear, indicating their acute inflammatory nature. However, this enhancement then disappears over the course of ensuing weeks to produce a typical hyperintense appearance on T2-weighted MRI scans. Only approximately 1 in 20 of the lesions visible on MRI result in an acute clinical episode, so that if a patient presents with what appears as an isolated syndrome, such as optic neuritis, a brain stem syndrome, or transverse myelitis causing bladder dysfunction, brain MRI is likely to show several cerebral lesions if the patient has multiple sclerosis. A change and increase in the number of lesions on MRI over the course of the next few months is now sufficient to secure a diagnosis of multiple sclerosis, according to the "McDonald criteria." This determination requires MRI or clinical evidence of dissemination in time and space.[43]

Very significant advances have been made in the past 15 years in understanding of the pathology of multiple sclerosis and possible treatments. Formerly thought of as a condition characterized by episodic central nervous system demyelination followed by a variable degree of remyelination, it has now become apparent that axonal loss is a prominent feature of this disease, resulting in spinal cord and brain atrophy.[44] Axonal loss starts early, probably soon after the first clinical episode when areas of demyelination are so highly visible on MRI scan.[45] Axonal loss is being increasingly recognized as the pathology that underlies the progressive nature of multiple sclerosis and leads to the accumulating neurologic deficits that characterize the illness.[46]

The sustained disability of Expanded Disability Status Scale (EDSS) level 4 (at which patients can walk approximately 500 m without aid or rest) is thought to herald the onset of secondary progressive multiple sclerosis and reflects the burden of axonal injury.[47] The mean time from EDSS level 4 to 6 (when there is intermittent or constant assistance required to walk 100 m) has been estimated to be 6 to 8.4 years[47–49] irrespective of any factors that at the onset may have been regarded as indicative of a good prognosis.

Bladder dysfunction mainly occurs in the presence of spinal cord involvement, which can either be part of an acute relapse, or with the accumulating deficit that characterizes progressive forms of the disease. There is a strong clinical impression that the measures needed to treat bladder dysfunction become increasingly demanding as spinal cord dysfunction increases and mobility deteriorates. Although patients may present with bladder dysfunction early in the disease if the initial clinically isolated syndrome is from a spinal cord lesion,[50] bladder dysfunction generally is related to the duration of multiple sclerosis[51] and degree of pyramidal symptoms in the lower limbs.[52,53] During the period of inexorable progression, bladder management may become particularly difficult, but the surgical options successfully applied to patients after traumatic spinal cord injury will prove unsuitable for those with deteriorating neurologic function. It is in this situation that detrusor injection of botulinum toxin has been proven to be so efficacious.[54]

In terms of treatment of the underlying neurologic disease, very significant progress has been made in the past 15 years, and now several effective treatments for multiple sclerosis are available. In 1995, the interferons were the first therapeutic agents shown to significantly modulate the immune response, and reduced the relapse rate by 30%.[55,56] Unfortunately, none of these agents nor copaxone, introduced at a similar time,[57] were highly effective in delaying the onset of significant neurologic deficit. All of these agents are administered through intramuscular or subcutaneous injections.

In 2003, a monoclonal antibody, adhesion molecule inhibitor, was shown to reduce relapse rate by 67%[58,59]; however, the development of progressive, multifocal leukoencephalopathy (PML) in patients receiving natalizumab temporarily suspended clinical trials and subsequent treatments. PML is a rare, progressive demyelinating disease of the central nervous system that may be fatal. It is caused by activation of JC virus, which usually remains latent and typically only causes PML in immunocompromised patients. The factors leading to activation of the latent infection are not fully understood. JC virus is widespread and the prevalence of antibodies increases with age. Among patients with multiple sclerosis receiving natalizumab, 31 cases of PML have been reported worldwide, 8 of which were fatal.[60] The reporting rate is equivalent to approximately one to two cases of PML for every 1000 patients treated with natalizumab for 2 or more years. Natalizumab should be promptly discontinued if PML is suspected, with subsequent appropriate evaluation, including a standardized MRI scan and lumbar puncture. Plasma exchange has been used to reduce natalizumab levels more quickly when PML has been identified.

Very recently two oral agents, cladribine and fingolomid, were shown to be effective in reducing relapse rates by more than 50%. Significant side effects include lymphopenia and herpes zoster virus; three cases of cancer for cladribine; and skin cancer and encephalitis in people taking fingolimod.[61,62] At the time of writing, it seems likely that these agents will soon become first-line treatment at the onset of multiple sclerosis.

Also now undergoing clinical trials is a new monoclonal antibody, alemtuzumab, which in phase II studies was shown to dramatically reduce relapse rate and disability scores, and prevent neurologic progression if given sufficiently early in the course of the illness.[63] However, this medication is not without potentially serious adverse events, and clinical trials were suspended in 2004 after one fatal case of immune thrombocytopenic purpura. Strategies have been put in place to monitor for this adverse event, which remains a risk. Additionally, 22.6% patients developed thyroid disease, which may require lifelong treatment.

Thus, in the future people with multiple sclerosis likely will be offered effective treatments very early in the course of their disease before the development of significant disability, but at a cost: the risk of developing potentially devastating side effects. With the long-term goal of preventing progression and disability, patients with multiple sclerosis undergoing treatment will require careful monitoring and a high level of clinical vigilance.

REFERENCES

1. Fowler CJ, Panicker JN, Emmanuel A, et al, editors. Pelvic organ dysfunction in neurological disease. Cambridge: Cambridge University Press; 2010.

2. Wein AJ, Kavoussi LR, Novick AC, et al, editors. Campbell-Walsh urology review manual. 3rd edition. Amsterdam: Saunders Elsevier; 2010.
3. Andrew J, Nathan PW. Lesions on the anterior frontal lobes and disturbances of micturition and defaecation. Brain 1964;87:233–62.
4. Fowler CJ, Griffiths DJ. A decade of functional brain imaging applied to bladder control. Neurourol Urodyn 2010;29(1):49–55.
5. Holstege G, Bandler R, Saper CB. The emotional motor system. Prog Brain Res 1996;107:3–6.
6. Griffiths D, Tadic SD. Bladder control, urgency, and urge incontinence: evidence from functional brain imaging. Neurourol Urodyn 2008;27(6):466–74.
7. Fowler CJ, Griffiths D, de Groat WC. The neural control of micturition. Nat Rev Neurosci 2008;9(6): 453–66.
8. Craig AD. How do you feel? Interoception: the sense of the physiological condition of the body. Nat Rev Neurosci 2002;3(8):655–66.
9. Milsom I, Abrams P, Cardozo L, et al. How widespread are the symptoms of an overactive bladder and how are they managed? A population-based prevalence study. BJU Int 2001;87(9):760–6.
10. Stewart WF, Van Rooyen JB, Cundiff GW, et al. Prevalence and burden of overactive bladder in the United States. World J Urol 2003;20(6):327–36.
11. Inouye SK, Studenski S, Tinetti ME, et al. Geriatric syndromes: clinical, research, and policy implications of a core geriatric concept. J Am Geriatr Soc 2007;55(5):780–91.
12. Kuo HK, Lipsitz LA. Cerebral white matter changes and geriatric syndromes: is there a link? J Gerontol A Biol Sci Med Sci 2004;59(8):818–26.
13. Sakakibara R, Hattori T, Uchiyama T, et al. Urinary function in elderly people with and without leukoaraiosis: relation to cognitive and gait function. J Neurol Neurosurg Psychiatry 1999;67(5):658–60.
14. Poggesi A, Pracucci G, Chabriat H, et al. Urinary complaints in nondisabled elderly people with age-related white matter changes: the Leukoaraiosis And DISability (LADIS) Study. J Am Geriatr Soc 2008;56(9):1638–43.
15. Kuchel GA, Moscufo N, Guttmann CR, et al. Localization of brain white matter hyperintensities and urinary incontinence in community-dwelling older adults. J Gerontol A Biol Sci Med Sci 2009;64(8): 902–9.
16. Gilman S, Wenning GK, Low PA, et al. Second consensus statement on the diagnosis of multiple system atrophy. Neurology 2008;71(9):670–6.
17. Yamamoto T, Sakakibara R, Uchiyama T, et al. Questionnaire-based assessment of pelvic organ dysfunction in multiple system atrophy. Mov Disord 2009;24(7):972–8.
18. Sakakibara R, Hattori T, Uchiyama T, et al. Videourodynamic and sphincter motor unit potential analyses in Parkinson's disease and multiple system atrophy. J Neurol Neurosurg Psychiatry 2001;71(5):600–6.
19. Benarroch EE, Schmeichel AM, Low PA, et al. Involvement of medullary serotonergic groups in multiple system atrophy. Ann Neurol 2004;55(3): 418–22.
20. Yoshida M. Multiple system atrophy: alpha-synuclein and neuronal degeneration. Neuropathology 2007; 27(5):484–93.
21. Ito T, Sakakibara R, Yasuda K, et al. Incomplete emptying and urinary retention in multiple-system atrophy: when does it occur and how do we manage it? Mov Disord 2006;21(6):816–23.
22. Hahn K, Ebersbach G. Sonographic assessment of urinary retention in multiple system atrophy and idiopathic Parkinson's disease. Mov Disord 2005;20 (11):1499–502.
23. Kirby RS, Fowler CJ, Gosling J, et al. Urethro-vesical dysfunction in progressive autonomic failure with multiple system atrophy. J Neurol Neurosurg Psychiatry 1986;49:554–62.
24. Mashidori T, Yamanishi T, Yoshida K, et al. Continuous urinary incontinence presenting as the initial symptoms demonstrating acontractile detrusor and intrinsic sphincter deficiency in multiple system atrophy. Int J Urol 2007;14(10):972–4.
25. Sakakibara R, Uchiyama T, Yamanishi T, et al. Bladder and bowel dysfunction in Parkinson's disease. J Neural Transm 2008;115(3):443–60.
26. Palace J, Chandiramani VA, Fowler CJ. Value of sphincter electromyography in the diagnosis of multiple system atrophy. Muscle Nerve 1997;20 (11):1396–403.
27. Tison F, Arne P, Sourgen C, et al. The value of external anal sphincter electromyography for the diagnosis of multiple system atrophy. Mov Disord 2000;15(6):1148–57.
28. Giladi N, Simon ES, Korczyn AD, et al. Anal sphincter EMG does not distinguish between multiple system atrophy and Parkinson's disease. Muscle Nerve 2000;23:731–4.
29. Paviour DC, Williams D, Fowler CJ, et al. Is sphincter electromyography a helpful investigation in the diagnosis of multiple system atrophy? A retrospective study with pathological diagnosis. Mov Disord 2005;20(11):1425–30.
30. Chaudhuri KR, Martinez-Martin P, Schapira AH, et al. International multicenter pilot study of the first comprehensive self-completed nonmotor symptoms questionnaire for Parkinson's disease: the NMSQuest study. Mov Disord 2006;21(7):916–23.
31. Martinez-Martin P, Schapira AH, Stocchi F, et al. Prevalence of nonmotor symptoms in Parkinson's disease in an international setting; Study using nonmotor symptoms questionnaire in 545 patients. Mov Disord 2007;22(11):1623–9.

32. Sakakibara R, Shinotoh H, Uchiyama T, et al. Questionnaire-based assessment of pelvic organ dysfunction in Parkinson's disease. Auton Neurosci 2001;92(1–2):76–85.
33. de Groat WC. Integrative control of the lower urinary tract: preclinical perspective. Br J Pharmacol 2006; 147(Suppl 2):S25–40.
34. Seki S, Igawa Y, Kaidoh K, et al. Role of Dopamine D1 and D1 receptors in the micturition reflex in conscious rats. Neurourol Urodyn 2001;20(1): 105–13.
35. Hineno T, Mizobuchi M, Hiratani K, et al. Disappearance of circadian rhythms in Parkinson's disease model induced by 1-methyl-4-phenyl-1,2,3,6-tetrahydropyridine in dogs. Brain Res 1992;580(1–2): 92–9.
36. Stocchi F, Carbone A, Inghilleri M, et al. Urodynamic and neurophysiological evaluation in Parkinson's disease and multiple system atrophy. J Neurol Neurosurg Psychiatry 1997;62:507–11.
37. Wheeler JS Jr, Siroky MB, Pavlakis AJ, et al. The changing neurourologic pattern of multiple sclerosis. J Urol 1983;130:1123–6.
38. Sakakibara R, Uchiyama T, Yamanishi T, et al. Genitourinary dysfunction in Parkinson's disease. Mov Disord 2010;25(1):2–12.
39. Braak H, Ghebremedhin E, Rüb U, et al. Stages in the development of Parkinson's disease-related pathology. Cell Tissue Res 2004;318(1):121–34.
40. Braak H, Rub U, Gai WP, et al. Idiopathic Parkinson's disease: possible routes by which vulnerable neuronal types may be subject to neuroinvasion by an unknown pathogen. J Neural Transm 2003;110 (5):517–36.
41. Staskin DS, Vardi Y, Siroky MB, et al. Post-prostatectomy incontinence in the parkinsonian patient: the significance of poor voluntary sphincter control. J Urol 1988;140:117–8.
42. Roth B, Studer UE, Fowler CJ, et al. Benign prostatic obstruction and Parkinson's disease—should transurethral resection of the prostate be avoided? J Urol 2009;181(5):2209–13.
43. Polman CH, Reingold SC, Edan G, et al. Diagnostic criteria for multiple sclerosis: 2005 revisions to the "McDonald Criteria". Ann Neurol 2005;58(6): 840–6.
44. Trapp BD, Peterson J, Ransohoff RM, et al. Axonal transection in the lesions of multiple sclerosis. N Engl J Med 1998;338(5):278–85.
45. Brex PA, Jenkins R, Fox NC, et al. Detection of ventricular enlargement in patients at the earliest clinical stage of MS. Neurology 2000;54(8): 1689–91.
46. Coles AJ, Cox A, Le Page E, et al. The window of therapeutic opportunity in multiple sclerosis: evidence from monoclonal antibody therapy. J Neurol 2006;253(1):98–108.
47. Confavreux C, Vukusic S, Moreau T, et al. Relapses and progression of disability in multiple sclerosis. N Engl J Med 2000;343(20):1430–8.
48. Confavreux C, Aimard G, Devic M, et al. Course and prognosis of multiple sclerosis assessed by the computerized data processing of 349 patients. Brain 1980;103(2):281–300.
49. Confavreux C, Vukusic S, Adeleine P, et al. Early clinical predictors and progression of irreversible disability in multiple sclerosis: an amnesic process. Brain 2003;126(Pt 4):770–82.
50. Kalita J, Shah S, Kapoor R, et al. Bladder dysfunction in acute transverse myelitis: magnetic resonance imaging and neurophysiological and urodynamic correlations. J Neurol Neurosurg Psychiatry 2002;73(2):154–9.
51. Awad SA, Gajewski JB, Sogbein SK, et al. Relationship between neurological and urological status in patients with multiple sclerosis. J Urol 1984;132: 499–502.
52. Betts CD, D'Mellow MT, Fowler CJ, et al. Urinary symptoms and the neurological features of bladder dysfunction in multiple sclerosis. J Neurol Neurosurg Psychiatry 1993;56:245–50.
53. Fowler CJ, Panicker JN, Drake M, et al. A UK consensus on the management of the bladder in multiple sclerosis. J Neurol Neurosurg Psychiatry 2009;80(5):470–7.
54. Kalsi V, Gonzales G, Popat R, et al. Botulinum injections for the treatment of bladder symptoms of multiple sclerosis. Ann Neurol 2007;62(5): 452–7.
55. Jacobs LD, Cookfair DL, Rudick RA, et al. Intramuscular interferon beta-1a for disease progression in relapsing multiple sclerosis. The Multiple Sclerosis Collaborative Research Group (MSCRG). Ann Neurol 1996;39(3):285–94.
56. Paty DW, Li DK. Interferon beta-lb is effective in relapsing-remitting multiple sclerosis. II. MRI analysis results of a multicenter, randomized, double-blind, placebo-controlled trial. 1993 [classical article]. Neurology 2001;57(12 Suppl 5):S10–5.
57. Comi G, Filippi M, Wolinsky JS, et al. European/ Canadian multicenter, double-blind, randomized, placebo-controlled study of the effects of glatiramer acetate on magnetic resonance imaging–measured disease activity and burden in patients with relapsing multiple sclerosis. European/Canadian Glatiramer Acetate Study Group. Ann Neurol 2001; 49(3):290–7.
58. Miller DH, Khan OA, Sheremata WA, et al. A controlled trial of natalizumab for relapsing multiple sclerosis. N Engl J Med 2003;348(1):15–23.
59. Polman CH, O'Connor PW, Havrdova E, et al. A randomized, placebo-controlled trial of natalizumab for relapsing multiple sclerosis. N Engl J Med 2006; 354(9):899–910.

60. Clifford D, DeLuca A, Simpson DM, et al. Natalizumab-associated progressive multifocal leukoencephalopathy in patients with multiple sclerosis: lessons from 28 cases. Lancet Neurol 2010;9(4):438–46.
61. Giovannoni G, Comi G, Cook S, et al. A placebo-controlled trial of oral cladribine for relapsing multiple sclerosis. N Engl J Med 2010;362(5):416–26.
62. Kappos L, Radue EW, O'Connor P, et al. A placebo-controlled trial of oral fingolimod in relapsing multiple sclerosis. N Engl J Med 2010;362(5):387–401.
63. Coles AJ, Compston DA, Selmaj KW, et al. Alemtuzumab vs. interferon beta-1a in early multiple sclerosis. N Engl J Med 2008;359(17):1786–801.

Management Goals for the Spina Bifida Neurogenic Bladder: A Review from Infancy to Adulthood

Arthur Mourtzinos, MD[a], John T. Stoffel, MD[b,*]

KEYWORDS

- Spina bifida • Myelomeningocele • Urinary incontinence
- Urological evaluation and therapy

Myelodysplasia, also commonly known as spina bifida, is a general term that describes incomplete closure of the vertebral column and malformation of the embryonic neural tube. This condition is associated with a prenatal folate deficiency and may occur more frequently in genetically susceptible individuals or mothers exposed to hyperthermia during pregnancy.[1,2] Although the estimated occurrence is 1 per 1000 births, the rate of spina bifida and anencephaly in the United States has been decreasing since the Federal Drug Administration mandated folate supplements to enriched grain products in 1998.[3]

Spina bifida malformations fall into 3 general categories:

Spina bifida occulta: In this type, incomplete closure of the lumbar vertebrae is minor and the spinal cord contents do not protrude through the defect. Clinical signs include a skin abnormality over the vertebral defect, such as a mole, hair, or dimple. The estimated prevalence of spina bifida occulta is 12% in an otherwise healthy population.[4] The condition is usually asymptomatic but can occasionally present with urinary pathologic conditions.[5,6]

Meningocele: In this type, the meninges protrude through a vertebral canal defect but the neural elements of the cord remain confined within the canal. This type of herniation usually occurs posterior to the spine, but anterior herniation can also occasionally occur, particularly along the sacrum.[7] Magnetic resonance imaging (MRI) is usually needed to identify the extent of the lesion.[8] Patients with meningocele may exhibit a wide range of neurologic symptoms depending on the location of the defect.

Myelomeningocele (MMC): In this type, neural roots or segments of the spinal cord herniate through the incompletely closed vertebrae. When fatty tissues are protruding in addition to cord structures, the condition is subgrouped as a lipomyelomeningocele. MMC accounts for most of the myelodysplasia diagnoses, and the pathologic condition usually occurs in the lumbar or sacral region. Patients with lesions in the sacrum are frequently able to ambulate, whereas patients with lesions in the higher level have increasing probability of loss of lower extremity function. In addition, many children with MMC have

[a] Department of Urology, Lahey Clinic, Tufts University School of Medicine, 41 Mall Road, Burlington, MA 01805, USA
[b] Department of Urology, Lahey Clinic, 41 Mall Road, Burlington, MA 01805, USA
* Corresponding author.
E-mail address: John_t_stoffel@lahey.org

Urol Clin N Am 37 (2010) 527–535
doi:10.1016/j.ucl.2010.06.009

urologic.theclinics.com

associated cerebellar tonsil herniation (Arnold-Chiari malformation) and are at risk for mental compromise. In one retrospective series from 1975, 52% of patients with MMC with lesions above the L2 vertebra had mean IQ scores less than 70.[9]

MANAGEMENT OF PEDIATRIC MMC URINARY PATHOLOGIC CONDITIONS

Urological care is initiated soon after a child with MMC is born and is maintained throughout childhood. The goals of pediatric MMC urinary management can be roughly divided into (1) preservation of renal function and (2) promoting urinary continence.

Preservation of Renal Function

Untreated urinary storage and emptying pathologies in children with MMC can affect long-term renal function.[10,11] Neurogenic bladder pathologies that commonly occur in patients with MMC include an elevated detrusor leak point pressure, vesicoureteral reflux (VUR), and detrusor–external sphincter dyssynergia (DSD). McGuire and colleagues[12] first showed increased risk for upper tract dilation in children with MMC with detrusor leak point pressures greater than 40 cm H_2O. VUR, particularly in female patients with MMC, has been shown to be a significant risk factor for renal compromise when associated with febrile urinary tract infections.[13–15] DSD, if present, may cause or exacerbate elevated detrusor leak point pressures and VUR. In assessing 188 children with MMC using urodynamics, van Gool and colleagues[16] noted bladder–external sphincter dyssynergy (with or without bladder overactivity) in 59% of children and found these children at a greater risk for having an elevated detrusor leak point pressure, low bladder compliance, and more severe reflux. Other investigators have also demonstrated these findings.[17]

However, in children with spina bifida, neurologic lesions are not always stable and bladder pathologies change. Spindel and colleagues[18] noted that 37% of 79 infants with MMC experienced external sphincter changes during the first 3 years of life, with the greatest number of changes occurring during the first year. Because urodynamic findings frequently change during longitudinal follow-up, serial urodynamic and upper tract evaluations are recommended every 6 months.[19] Neurologic and urological changes may also occur because of a tethered cord. Fone and colleagues[20] examined the outcome of tethered cord release on preoperative bladder pathologies on 28 patients with MMC and found improved detrusor overactivity or bladder compliance in 30% and worse urodynamic patterns in 48% of the patients. Only 14% of patients experienced improved urinary control after the procedure. Consequently, because preoperative urodynamics do not seem to predict urological outcome of tethered cord release,[21,22] urodynamics and upper tract testing need to be performed at regular intervals after cord release to ensure bladder and upper tract safety.

Treatment plans for renal protection in patients with MMC have changed over the years. In the past, many children with MMC with voiding dysfunction were immediately treated with urinary diversion to preserve renal function. Shapiro and colleagues[23] published 10-year outcomes on 90 children with MMC treated with ileal loop diversion and showed stable renal units in 69% of the patients. However, other investigators found increasing morbidity with diversions over time.[24,25] Contemporary management for children with MMC with neurogenic bladder pathologies now focuses on lowering the urinary storage pressures with anticholinergic medication and avoiding elevated voiding pressures through clean intermittent catheterization (CIC). Using these principles, Kasabian and colleagues[26] demonstrated normal renal function in 92% of children with MMC with voiding dysfunction treated with oxybutynin and CIC. Other investigators have noted a decreased need for surgical intervention among children with MMC treated with anticholinergics and CIC. Kochakarn and colleagues[11] compared Thai children who were started on CIC at a mean of 7 months against a group of children started at a mean of 45 months and found that 27% and 14% of the early treatment group had hydronephrosis and underwent cystoplasty when compared with 58% and 32% in the late treatment group. However, investigators note that the efficacy of anticholinergic and CIC therapy needs to be monitored through urodynamics and patients followed up with only radiological evaluations may be at particularly high risk for upper tract compromise.[27]

Despite the advances in behavioral and pharmacologic therapies, some children with MMC progress to urinary reconstruction for renal protection. Autoaugmentation (resection of the detrusor while maintaining mucosal integrity) has been attempted to improve urinary storage pressure, although outcomes have been inconsistent. Dik and colleagues[28] evaluated 35 patients treated with autoaugmentation and noted improved bladder compliance in 16 and improved capacity in 13 patients. In contrast, MacNeily and colleagues[29] reported a 71% failure rate for upper tract protection and treatment of incontinence in a series of 17 patients with MMC. Enterocystoplasty is a more common treatment for refractory bladder pressures greater than 40 cm H_2O. In an epidemiologic study of Children's Hospitals, 12,925 unique spina bifida cases were examined, and 5% of these children underwent enterocystoplasty.[30] However, in a review of 226 studies on enterocystoplasty in patients with spina bifida, Scales and Weiner[31] noted that enterocystoplasty outcomes were difficult to compare between institutions because investigators do not use consistent posttreatment endpoints. Despite these comparative limitations, multiple studies show that children with MMC treated with enterocystoplasty experience long-term renal stability and resolution of VUR.[31–33]

Appendicovesicostomy or other continent urinary stoma procedures may also be performed to aid the neurologically compromised patient with MMC in performing CIC. Occasionally, the Malone antegrade continence enema procedure can be used to address concomitant bowel and urinary problems for the symptomatic patient with MMC. Hensle and colleagues[34] reported good bowel and urinary continence with this technique, although the number of urinary stomal complications were significant.

Promoting Urinary Continence

Urodynamic studies have demonstrated a high rate of detrusor overactivity, DSD, and sphincteric incompetence in children with MMC, often resulting in involuntary urinary leakage.[16] For children with MMC with DSD and detrusor overactivity, incontinence is treated by maximally relaxing the bladder with anticholinergics and then draining urine through CIC. Complications from this regimen are relatively uncommon, and CIC does not seem to greatly increase the risk of febrile urinary tract infections when compared with a sterile catheterization technique.[26,35] Campbell and colleagues[36] retrospectively reviewed CIC-related complications in patients with MMC and found an incidence of only 3.5 complications per 1000 patient-years. However, CIC can greatly affect family dynamics, and studies have shown decreased caregiver quality of life for patients with MMC treated with this technique.[37] Similar to CIC anticholinergics are generally well tolerated, but Ferrara and colleagues[38] noted a higher complication rate when the medication is given orally than in an intravesical route.

Botulinum toxin injections are a developing therapy for patients with MMC with urinary incontinence/retention from detrusor overactivity and sphincter dyssynergia, although there are few large series examining treatment efficacy. In one of the larger series, Akbar and colleagues[39] reported outcomes in 19 children with MMC treated with 20 U/kg body weight of Dysport botulinum toxin A and noted significant improvements in bladder compliance, maximum detrusor pressure, and maximum bladder capacity over a 4.5-year follow-up. More research is needed to determine how botulinum toxin can be optimally used for the population with MMC.

Some children with MMC with symptomatic urinary incontinence caused by sphincteric incompetence may benefit from surgical reconstruction of the bladder outlet. Good outcomes have been reported with multiple techniques, such as suburethral or wraparound slings[40] and bladder neck reconstructions or lengthening.[41] Artificial urinary sphincters can also be used to treat sphincteric incompetence in children with MMC, and long-term data suggest reasonable efficacy but a relatively high complication rate. Kryger and colleagues[42] reported that 13 of 47 children had sphincteric erosion or infection requiring explantation during a mean 15.4-year follow-up. Risk factors for erosion included previous erosion, prior bladder neck surgery, and a reservoir pressure greater than 70 cm H_2O. In addition, in their series of 30 patients who were followed up over a mean period of 6.5 years, Spiess and colleagues[43] noted that artificial urinary sphincter implantation rarely lasted longer than 8 years before requiring explantation. Endoscopic bulking agents have also been used to treat stress incontinence in children with MMC, although efficacy and duration of these agents are somewhat limited.[44]

However, surgeons need to consider the possibility that tightening the bladder outlet in children with MMC may increase the risk for upper tract compromise in selected patients.[45] Investigators have reported successful sling placement in selected children with MMC without compromising storage or voiding pressures. Austin and colleagues[40] reported outcomes in 18 children with MMC treated with slings and found little change in detrusor leak point pressure after surgery (23.2 cm H_2O both before and after). Likewise, Snodgrass and colleagues[46] reported no detrimental urodynamic changes after bladder neck sling placement in children with MMC with preoperative detrusor pressures less than 25 cm H_2O. However, Lopez Pereira and colleagues[47] noted in their series that 31% of children undergoing artificial urinary sphincter placement developed significant physiologic changes in the bladder and ultimately required enterocystoplasty.

ADOLESCENT ISSUES

There is concern among practitioners that prostatic growth in male patients or estrogenization of the urethra in female patients during puberty may cause increased outlet resistance, which could then increase bladder pressures and place the upper tract at risk. Almodhen and colleagues[48] evaluated 37 children with MMC treated conservatively and they found that puberty was associated with an increase in maximum cystometric capacity, detrusor pressure, and detrusor leak point pressure. However, no significant change in upper tract function was noted within this small population. There are few other studies that examine whether puberty does indeed increase risk of upper tract compromise in patients with MMC.

Many children with MMC also develop increasing concerns over body image as puberty approaches. Appleton and colleagues[49] noted a relationship between body image and an increased propensity toward depression in adolescents with MMC, although depression is mitigated by a higher level of perceived parental social support. Concerns over body image or alternations in mood may cause decreased patient compliance in following CIC regimens, taking prescribed medications, or maintaining urological follow-up. Studies have shown that patients with spina bifida with urinary incontinence are at an even greater risk for lower self-esteem, particularly female patients.[50] Consequently, urologists should attempt every effort to maintain regular follow-up schedules with children with MMC during adolescence so that incontinence issues can be addressed.

Sexual issues can become more prominent for patients with MMC during adolescence, particularly in male patients. In an assessment of 121 adolescents and young adults with MMC, women with MMC were 2.3 times more likely to be sexually active than men with MMC.[51] This disparity is likely caused by the high prevalence of erectile dysfunction among men with MMC. Diamond and colleagues[52] reviewed the neuroanatomy of 52 postpubertal men with MMC and found that only 14% of patients with lesions above T10 region and negative anocutaneous reflex could achieve erections. In addition, in a survey of 157 adolescent and young adult patients with spina bifida (age range 16–25 years), Verhoef and colleagues[53] found that only 52% were satisfied with their sexual lives. Urinary incontinence, low self-confidence, and a history of hydrocephalus were identified as risk factors for lower sexual functioning. From this study it was concluded that sexual consoling should be included as part of regular adolescent urological care. Overgoor and colleagues[54] reported successful treatment of erectile dysfunction in 3 patients with spina bifida with lumbar lesions by anastomosing the sensory ilioinguinal nerve to the ipsilateral dorsal nerve of the penis. More research will determine if techniques such as these offer long-term improvement for erectile dysfunction in patients with spina bifida.

TRANSITION TO ADULTHOOD

As a result of advances in medical care, children with MMC are now surviving to adulthood in greater numbers. However, mortality still remains high. Oakshott and colleagues[55] consecutively followed up 117 patients with spina bifida who were born between 1963 and 1971 and found that 33% of patients died before the age of 5 years and an additional 26% died over the next 35 years. Most common causes of death included epilepsy, pulmonary embolus, acute hydrocephalus, and acute renal sepsis. Mortality was particularly high in patients with neurologic lesions above T11 region. One possible reason for the increased mortality is that although care for the pediatric patient with MMC is carefully coordinated through urologists, neurosurgeons, orthopedic surgeons, primary care physicians, and social workers, once patients with MMC leave pediatric care or transition to independent living, many fail to reestablish regular follow-up. A study suggested that up to two-thirds of adults with spina bifida do not routinely seek regular urological follow-up.[56] Consequently, it is recommended that adolescents begin the complex process of understanding their unique urological treatment plan and actively participate in establishing adult care.[57]

RECOMMENDED ROUTINE UROLOGICAL EVALUATIONS FOR ADULTS WITH SPINA BIFIDA

Upper Tract Surveillance

There are no formal urological recommendations or guidelines regarding upper tract surveillance for adults with MMC. Most neurourologists recommend a yearly renal ultrasonography and serum creatinine level measurement in patients with a neurogenic bladder, particularly if there is a history of lower urinary tract reconstructive surgery.[58–60] In the absence of known upper tract pathology, ultrasonography is generally preferable because there is no radiation exposure. However, computed tomography (CT) urograms or intravenous pyelograms may be needed for evaluation of hematuria, recurrent urinary tract infections, pyelonephritis, stones, or if an abnormality is detected on routine ultrasonography. At the authors' institution, voiding cystourethrography and nuclear medicine renal function scans are also performed yearly for patients with MMC and an unresolved history of VUR or progressive renal compromise.

Bladder Physiology

Bladders of adult patients with MMC should not be considered stable during the transition from childhood through adolescence and then into adulthood. Baseline video urodynamics in the adult patient should be obtained after the first visit. Although a simple cystometrography is useful in determining detrusor overactivity and Valsalva leak point pressures, the patient's bladder compliance and detrusor leak point pressures may be underestimated if there is concomitant VUR or bladder diverticuli. In a review of the data from 257 consecutive unselected patients undergoing video urodynamics in the authors' institution, those with a bladder compliance less than 20 $cm^3/cm\ H_2O$ were 4.3 times more likely to have a finding of bladder diverticuli or VUR on concomitant fluoroscopy compared with patients with compliance greater than 20 $cm^3/cm\ H_2O$ ($P<.001$) (Stoffel JT, unpublished data, 2006). Consequently, the authors recommend video-urodynamic testing for MMC baseline evaluation.

As with upper tract imaging, there are no standardized recommendations for the timing of urodynamic testing. New symptoms such as unexpected urinary continence, increased leakage between catheterization, and persistent urinary tract infections should prompt a urodynamic evaluation. Likewise, symptom changes in the setting of new musculoskeletal findings should also prompt performing an MRI to assess for a tethered cord. At the authors' institution, it is attempted to perform urodynamics annually for adults with MMC and with elevated bladder storage pressures or a history of hydronephrosis/decreased glomerular filtration. For asymptomatic patients with stable tracts, urodynamics are performed every 2 to 3 years.

Cancer Surveillance

There is some evidence to suggest that patients with spina bifida are at higher risk for developing aggressive cancers of the urothelium at a younger age. In the series by Austin and colleagues[61] of 8 patients with spina bifida with bladder malignancies, the mean patient age was 41 years, and 88% of the patients presented with pathologic T3 stage or greater stage. Median survival was 6 months. Only 1 of 8 patients had a previous augmentation cystoplasty, and all patients had experienced chronic urinary tract infections. Augmentation cystoplasty may also increase cancer risk for patients with MMC. Soergel and colleagues[62] reported a 1.2% incidence of bladder cancer in augmented bladders from children, assuming a 10-year lag period before the cancer risk matures. However, the absolute risk associated with augmentation is difficult to assess, given the high prevalence of confounding carcinogenic stimuli in this population. Given this unclear cancer risk in patients with MMC, yearly cytologic examination of urine and, if possible, cystoscopy are recommended.

ADDITIONAL ADULT UROLOGICAL SPINA BIFIDA CONCERNS

Persistent Urinary Incontinence

It is unclear if the successes in treating pediatric urinary incontinence continue into adulthood. Verhoef and colleagues[63] assessed urinary continence among patients with spina bifida in the Netherlands by surveying the number of patients with one or more bladder accidents in a month. Of the 179 patients with MMC, 60.9% reported urinary incontinence, regardless of the type of bladder management. Approximately 70% of the patients perceived urinary incontinence as a problem. Other series also report a high prevalence of adult MMC urinary incontinence. Lemelle and colleagues[64] reviewed the management of urinary incontinence in 421 patients with MMC, 191 (45%) of whom had been previously treated for urinary leakage. The average age of patients in this cohort was 21.7 years, and 65% of patients reported either continuous or frequent urinary leakage. Despite these reports, other investigators have reported successful treatment of adult MMC stress incontinence with fascia slings and urethral lengthening.[65] However, given the complexity of these patients, it is the authors' recommendation that a urologist should initiate a new workup with urodynamics, upper tract imaging, and cystoscopy before starting treatment for incontinence in an adult with MMC. Once the incontinence pathophysiology is understood, the appropriate treatment can be initiated.

Chronic Urinary Tract Infections

Patients with MMC remain at risk for chronic urinary tract infections. Dicianno and Wilson[66] reviewed the 2004-2005 data from the National Inpatient Sample for patients with MMC who are older than 18 years and found that the most common reason for admission was symptomatic urinary tract infections. In a different review, Kinsman and Doehring[67] noted that nearly 50% of MMC admissions were attributed to preventable causes such as urinary tract infections and stones. Although there are no guidelines for treating bacteriuria in patients with MMC, Elliott and colleagues[68] surveyed 59 spina bifida clinics and noted that most clinics treated patients with urine cultures positive for bacteria with more than 10^4 colony-forming units/mL when this finding was associated with fever, flank pain, dysuria, change in urinary patterns, or a white blood cell count greater than 50 on urinalysis. In addition to the above recommendations, the authors empirically treat patients with MMC with CIC or based on a history of urinary diversion when the patient reports a clinical change in urine odor or sediment over 24 hours. Urine cultures are performed in patients if they experience persistent urinary symptoms after 2 days of oral antibiotic treatment or if there is a history of urinary calculi or VUR.

Complications from Lower Urinary Tract Reconstruction

Children with MMC who undergo reconstructive bladder surgery to promote long-term renal health may experience complications that continue into adulthood. Rubenwolf and colleagues[69] reviewed surgical complications from a series of 44 children with neurogenic bladders (24 with MMC) treated with enterocystoplasty or continent urinary diversion. Although approximately 90% of the patients achieved stable upper tracts, 39% experienced stomal complications, stones formed in 19%, and ureteric stenosis in 8%. In other series, approximately 25% of continent urinary stoma procedures required revision.[70,71] Although it is the authors' practice to surgically correct compromised continent stomas, some adults with MMC may have additional medical comorbidities, making surgical correction prohibitive. In these situations, patients can be temporarily managed with a percutaneous cystostomy tube while medical issues such as obesity, hygiene, and decubitus ulcers are optimized.

Urologists should also consider additional complications related to urinary diversions or enterocystoplasty in patients with MMC who have underwent lower urinary tract reconstruction. Renal compromise may present over time, although Stein[72] reported outcomes on 149 children and young adults with urinary diversions/reconstructions and found upper tract stability in more than 95% over a 12-year follow-up. However, stones, infection, malabsorption, and failure to catheterize may cause significant morbidity.[73,74] Reservoir perforations can be a rare source of abdominal pain and morbidity for the augmented patient with MMC. Rushton and colleagues[75] reported on 4 patients with spina bifida presenting with bladder rupture 6 months to 3 years after enterocystoplasty. All patients were managed with intermittent catheterization, and 3 patients initially had normal cystograms on presentation. In general, the practicing urologist should have a low threshold to perform a CT cystography if bladder perforation is suspected.

SUMMARY

As children with spina bifida transition into adolescence and adulthood, they remain at risk for considerable urological morbidity. The urologist caring for the adult patient with spina bifida needs to be aware of pediatric treatment goals and should vigorously screen for developing upper and lower urinary tract pathologic conditions. With routine follow-up, the adult patient with spina bifida should enjoy a stable renal function, a reasonable level of urinary continence, and a high urological quality of life.

REFERENCES

1. Czeizel AE. Primary prevention of neural-tube defects and some other major congenital abnormalities: recommendations for the appropriate use of folic acid during pregnancy. Paediatr Drugs 2000;2(6):437–49.
2. Moretti ME, Bar-Oz B, Fried S, et al. Maternal hyperthermia and the risk for neural tube defects in offspring: systematic review and meta-analysis. Epidemiology 2005;16(2):216–9.
3. Boulet SL, Yang Q, Mai C, et al. Trends in the post-fortification prevalence of spina bifida and anencephaly in the United States. Birth Defects Res A Clin Mol Teratol 2008;82(7):527–32.
4. Eubanks JD, Cheruvu VK. Prevalence of sacral spina bifida occulta and its relationship to age, sex, race, and the sacral table angle: an anatomic, osteologic study of three thousand one hundred specimens. Spine (Phila Pa 1976) 2009;34(15):1539–43.
5. Sakakibara R, Hattori T, Uchiyama T, et al. Uroneurological assessment of spina bifida cystica and occulta. Neurourol Urodyn 2003;22(4):328–34.
6. Mandell J, Bauer SB, Hallett M, et al. Occult spinal dysraphism: a rare but detectable cause of voiding dysfunction. Urol Clin North Am 1980;7(2):349–56.
7. Van Allen MI. Multisite neural tube closure in humans. Birth Defects Orig Artic Ser 1996;30(1):203–25.

8. Tortori-Donati P, Rossi A, Biancheri R, et al. Magnetic resonance imaging of spinal dysraphism. Top Magn Reson Imaging 2001;12(6):375–409.
9. Shurtleff DB, Hayden PW, Chapman WH, et al. Problems of long-term survival and social function. West J Med 1975;122(3):199–205.
10. Dik P, Klijn AJ, van Gool JD, et al. Early start to therapy preserves kidney function in spina bifida patients. Eur Urol 2006;49(5):908–13.
11. Kochakarn W, Ratana-Olarn K, Lertsithichai P, et al. Follow-up of long-term treatment with clean intermittent catheterization for neurogenic bladder in children. Asian J Surg 2004;27(2):134–6.
12. McGuire EJ, Woodside JR, Borden TA, et al. Prognostic value of urodynamic testing in myelodysplastic patients. 1981. J Urol 2002;167(2 Pt 2):1049–53 [discussion: 1054].
13. DeLair SM, Eandi J, White MJ, et al. Renal cortical deterioration in children with spinal dysraphism: analysis of risk factors. J Spinal Cord Med 2007;30 (Suppl 1):S30–4.
14. Torre M, Buffa P, Jasonni V, et al. Long-term urologic outcome in patients with caudal regression syndrome, compared with meningomyelocele and spinal cord lipoma. J Pediatr Surg 2008;43(3):530–3.
15. Shiroyanagi Y, Suzuki M, Matsuno D, et al. The significance of 99mtechnetium dimercaptosuccinic acid renal scan in children with spina bifida during long-term followup. J Urol 2009;181(5):2262–6 [discussion: 2266].
16. van Gool JD, Dik P, de Jong TP. Bladder-sphincter dysfunction in myelomeningocele. Eur J Pediatr 2001;160(7):414–20.
17. Ozel SK, Dokumcu Z, Akyildiz C, et al. Factors affecting renal scar development in children with spina bifida. Urol Int 2007;79(2):133–6.
18. Spindel MR, Bauer SB, Dyro FM, et al. The changing neurourologic lesion in myelodysplasia. JAMA 1987;258(12):1630–3.
19. Roach MB, Switters DM, Stone AR. The changing urodynamic pattern in infants with myelomeningocele. J Urol 1993;150(3):944–7.
20. Fone PD, Vapnek JM, Litwiller SE, et al. Urodynamic findings in the tethered spinal cord syndrome: does surgical release improve bladder function? J Urol 1997;157(2):604–9.
21. Guerra LA, Pike J, Milks J, et al. Outcome in patients who underwent tethered cord release for occult spinal dysraphism. J Urol 2006;176(4 Pt 2):1729–32.
22. Macejko AM, Cheng EY, Yerkes EB, et al. Clinical urological outcomes following primary tethered cord release in children younger than 3 years. J Urol 2007;178(4 Pt 2):1738–42 [discussion: 1742–3].
23. Shapiro SR, Lebowitz R, Colodny AH. Fate of 90 children with ileal conduit urinary diversion a decade later: analysis of complications, pyelography, renal function and bacteriology. J Urol 1975;114(2):289–95.
24. Schwarz GR, Jeffs RD. Ileal conduit urinary diversion in children: computer analysis of followup from 2 to 16 years. J Urol 1975;114(2):285–8.
25. Cass AS, Luxenberg M, Johnson CF, et al. Management of the neurogenic bladder in 413 children. J Urol 1984;132(3):521–5.
26. Kasabian NG, Bauer SB, Dyro FM, et al. The prophylactic value of clean intermittent catheterization and anticholinergic medication in newborns and infants with myelodysplasia at risk of developing urinary tract deterioration. Am J Dis Child 1992;146(7):840–3.
27. Kaufman AM, Ritchey ML, Roberts AC, et al. Decreased bladder compliance in patients with myelomeningocele treated with radiological observation. J Urol 1996;156(6):2031–3.
28. Dik P, Tsachouridis GD, Klijn AJ, et al. Detrusorectomy for neuropathic bladder in patients with spinal dysraphism. J Urol 2003;170(4 Pt 1):1351–4.
29. MacNeily AE, Afshar K, Coleman GU, et al. Autoaugmentation by detrusor myotomy: its lack of effectiveness in the management of congenital neuropathic bladder. J Urol 2003;170(4 Pt 2):1643–6 [discussion: 1646].
30. Lendvay TS, Cowan CA, Mitchell MM, et al. Augmentation cystoplasty rates at children's hospitals in the United States: a pediatric health information system database study. J Urol 2006;176(4 Pt 2):1716–20.
31. Scales CD Jr, Wiener JS. Evaluating outcomes of enterocystoplasty in patients with spina bifida: a review of the literature. J Urol 2008;180(6):2323–9.
32. Singh G, Thomas DG. Enterocystoplasty in the neuropathic bladder. Neurourol Urodyn 1995;14(1):5–10.
33. Juhasz Z, Somogyi R, Vajda P, et al. Does the type of bladder augmentation influence the resolution of pre-existing vesicoureteral reflux? Urodynamic studies. Neurourol Urodyn 2008;27(5):412–6.
34. Hensle TW, Reiley EA, Chang DT. The Malone antegrade continence enema procedure in the management of patients with spina bifida. J Am Coll Surg 1998;186(6):669–74.
35. Joseph DB, Bauer SB, Colodny AH, et al. Clean, intermittent catheterization of infants with neurogenic bladder. Pediatrics 1989;84(1):78–82.
36. Campbell JB, Moore KN, Voaklander DC, et al. Complications associated with clean intermittent catheterization in children with spina bifida. J Urol 2004;171(6 Pt 1):2420–2.
37. Borzyskowski M, Cox A, Edwards M, et al. Neuropathic bladder and intermittent catheterization: social and psychological impact on families. Dev Med Child Neurol 2004;46(3):160–7.

38. Ferrara P, D'Aleo CM, Tarquini E, et al. Side-effects of oral or intravesical oxybutynin chloride in children with spina bifida. BJU Int 2001;87(7):674–8.
39. Akbar M, Abel R, Seyler TM, et al. Repeated botulinum-A toxin injections in the treatment of myelodysplastic children and patients with spinal cord injuries with neurogenic bladder dysfunction. BJU Int 2007;100(3):639–45.
40. Austin PF, Westney OL, Leng WW, et al. Advantages of rectus fascial slings for urinary incontinence in children with neuropathic bladders. J Urol 2001; 165(6 Pt 2):2369–71 [discussion: 2371–2].
41. Hayes MC, Bulusu A, Terry T, et al. The Pippi Salle urethral lengthening procedure; experience and outcome from three United Kingdom centres. BJU Int 1999;84(6):701–5.
42. Kryger JV, Spencer Barthold J, Fleming P, et al. The outcome of artificial urinary sphincter placement after a mean 15-year follow-up in a paediatric population. BJU Int 1999;83(9):1026–31.
43. Spiess PE, Capolicchio JP, Kiruluta G, et al. Is an artificial sphincter the best choice for incontinent boys with spina bifida? Review of our long term experience with the AS-800 artificial sphincter. Can J Urol 2002;9(2):1486–91.
44. Godbole P, Bryant R, MacKinnon AE, et al. Endourethral injection of bulking agents for urinary incontinence in children. BJU Int 2003;91(6):536–9.
45. Dave S, Pippi Salle JL, Lorenzo AJ, et al. Is long-term bladder deterioration inevitable following successful isolated bladder outlet procedures in children with neuropathic bladder dysfunction? J Urol 2008;179(5):1991–6 [discussion: 1996].
46. Snodgrass W, Barber T, Cost N. Detrusor compliance changes after bladder neck sling without augmentation in children with neurogenic urinary incontinence. J Urol 2010;183:2361–6.
47. Lopez Pereira P, Somoza Ariba I, Martinez Urrutia MJ, et al. Artificial urinary sphincter: 11-year experience in adolescents with congenital neuropathic bladder. Eur Urol 2006;50(5): 1096–101 [discussion: 1101].
48. Almodhen F, Capolicchio JP, Jednak R, et al. Postpubertal urodynamic and upper urinary tract changes in children with conservatively treated myelomeningocele. J Urol 2007;178(4 Pt 1):1479–82.
49. Appleton PL, Ellis NC, Minchom PE, et al. Depressive symptoms and self-concept in young people with spina bifida. J Pediatr Psychol 1997;22(5): 707–22.
50. Moore C, Kogan BA, Parekh A. Impact of urinary incontinence on self-concept in children with spina bifida. J Urol 2004;171(4):1659–62.
51. Cardenas DD, Topolski TD, White CJ, et al. Sexual functioning in adolescents and young adults with spina bifida. Arch Phys Med Rehabil 2008;89(1): 31–5.
52. Diamond DA, Rickwood AM, Thomas DG. Penile erections in myelomeningocele patients. Br J Urol 1986;58(4):434–5.
53. Verhoef M, Barf HA, Vroege JA, et al. Sex education, relationships, and sexuality in young adults with spina bifida. Arch Phys Med Rehabil 2005; 86(5):979–87.
54. Overgoor ML, Kon M, Cohen-Kettenis PT, et al. Neurological bypass for sensory innervation of the penis in patients with spina bifida. J Urol 2006;176(3):1086–90 [discussion: 1090].
55. Oakeshott P, Hunt GM, Poulton A, et al. Expectation of life and unexpected death in open spina bifida: a 40-year complete, non-selective, longitudinal cohort study. Dev Med Child Neurol 2010;52(8): 749–53.
56. Hunt GM. Open spina bifida: outcome for a complete cohort treated unselectively and followed into adulthood. Dev Med Child Neurol 1990;32(2):108–18.
57. Mukherjee S. Transition to adulthood in spina bifida: changing roles and expectations. ScientificWorldJournal 2007;7:1890–5.
58. Blok BF, Karsenty G, Corcos J. Urological surveillance and management of patients with neurogenic bladder: results of a survey among practicing urologists in Canada. Can J Urol 2006;13(5):3239–43.
59. Persun ML, Ginsberg PC, Harmon JD, et al. Role of urologic evaluation in the adult spina bifida patient. Urol Int 1999;62(4):205–8.
60. Razdan S, Leboeuf L, Meinbach DS, et al. Current practice patterns in the urologic surveillance and management of patients with spinal cord injury. Urology 2003;61(5):893–6.
61. Austin JC, Elliott S, Cooper CS. Patients with spina bifida and bladder cancer: atypical presentation, advanced stage and poor survival. J Urol 2007; 178(3 Pt 1):798–801.
62. Soergel TM, Cain MP, Misseri R, et al. Transitional cell carcinoma of the bladder following augmentation cystoplasty for the neuropathic bladder. J Urol 2004;172(4 Pt 2):1649–51 [discussion: 1651–2].
63. Verhoef M, Lurvink M, Barf HA, et al. High prevalence of incontinence among young adults with spina bifida: description, prediction and problem perception. Spinal Cord 2005;43(6):331–40.
64. Lemelle JL, Guillemin F, Aubert D, et al. A multicenter evaluation of urinary incontinence management and outcome in spina bifida. J Urol 2006;175(1):208–12.
65. Herschorn S, Radomski SB. Fascial slings and bladder neck tapering in the treatment of male neurogenic incontinence. J Urol 1992;147(4): 1073–5.
66. Dicianno BE, Wilson R. Hospitalizations of adults with spina bifida and congenital spinal cord anomalies. Arch Phys Med Rehabil 2010;91(4):529–35.

67. Kinsman SL, Doehring MC. The cost of preventable conditions in adults with spina bifida. Eur J Pediatr Surg 1996;6(Suppl 1):17–20.
68. Elliott SP, Villar R, Duncan B. Bacteriuria management and urological evaluation of patients with spina bifida and neurogenic bladder: a multicenter survey. J Urol 2005;173(1):217–20.
69. Rubenwolf PC, Beissert A, Gerharz EW, et al. 15 years of continent urinary diversion and enterocystoplasty in children and adolescents: the Wurzburg experience. BJU Int 2010;105(5):698–705.
70. Khair B, Azmy AF, Carachi R, et al. Continent urinary diversion using Mitrofanoff principle in children with neurogenic bladder. Eur J Pediatr Surg 1993;3 (Suppl 1):8–9.
71. Van der Aa F, Joniau S, De Baets K, et al. Continent catheterizable vesicostomy in an adult population: success at high costs. Neurourol Urodyn 2009;28(6):487–91.
72. Stein R, Fisch M, Ermert A, et al. Urinary diversion and orthotopic bladder substitution in children and young adults with neurogenic bladder: a safe option for treatment? J Urol 2000;163(2):568–73.
73. Woodhouse CR. Myelomeningocele in young adults. BJU Int 2005;95(2):223–30.
74. Fichtner J. Follow-up after urinary diversion. Urol Int 1999;63(1):40–5.
75. Rushton HG, Woodard JR, Parrott TS, et al. Delayed bladder rupture after augmentation enterocystoplasty. J Urol 1988;140(2):344–6.

Spinal Cord/Brain Injury and the Neurogenic Bladder

Seong Jin Jeong, MD[a], Sung Yong Cho, MD[b], Seung-June Oh, MD[b,*]

KEYWORDS

• Neurogenic bladder • Spinal cord injury
• Cerebrovascular accident • Traumatic brain injury
• Urodynamics • Disease management

The mortality of patients with neurogenic bladder (NB) secondary to major neurologic abnormalities has declined dramatically with improved care for NB. However, clinical studies on this condition are still relatively lacking. This article reviews NB related to traumatic injury as well as vascular lesion of spinal cord/brain.

MECHANICAL/TRAUMATIC INJURIES TO THE SPINAL CORD AND BRAIN

Although no accurate data on the overall incidence of spinal cord injury (SCI) have been obtained in the United States since 1970s,[1] a prevalence of more than 200,000 patients with traumatic SCI[2] has been estimated in the United States, with an incidence of approximately 12,000 patients being newly diagnosed with SCI every year.[1] The main causes of SCI are motor vehicle accidents (42.1%) and falls (26.7%).[1] On the other hand, more than 2 million individuals in the United States were admitted to the emergency room due to traumatic brain injury (TBI),[3] and about 50% of the patients suffered moderate to severe injuries. The predominant cause of TBI is fall. The possibility of concurrent SCI and TBI should always be considered when encountering a patient with SCI[4]: 11% of patients with SCI have an associated head injury.[2] TBI and SCI may result in different types of voiding dysfunction, and their coexistence can make accurate diagnosis challenging.

Expected Bladder Dysfunction by SCI Level

In principle, SCI above the S1 level does not interrupt the integrity of parasympathetic (S2 through S4) and somatic nerves (S1 through S4). Only cortical inhibition of voiding reflex and detrusor-sphincter coordination regulated by the pontine micturition center are disturbed.[5] Injury at the S2-S4 level can result in impairment of detrusor contractility and malfunction of pudendal nerves, which innervate the distal sphincter. Involuntary detrusor contraction (IDC) after an injury at the C2-S1 region and open fixed tone of the distal sphincter by denervation after S2-S4 injury can induce storage failure.[6] In addition, detrusor-sphincter dyssynergia (DSD) after C2-S1 injury and detrusor underactivity (DU)/detrusor acontractility (DA) or nonrelaxing urethral sphincter obstruction after S2-S4 injury can result in failure to empty.[7] Because the nuclei of the pelvic nerves involved in contraction of the detrusor muscle and the pudendal nerves responsible for contraction of the striated sphincter are located in different portions of the sacral cord (intermediolateral cell column vs ventral gray matter), sacral SCI can induce DA, leaving striated sphincter function intact.[2]

The authors have nothing to disclose.
[a] Department of Urology, Seoul National University Bundang Hospital, 300 Gumi-dong, Bundang-gu, Seongnam-si, Seongnam, 463-707, Korea
[b] Department of Urology, Seoul National University College of Medicine, Seoul National University Hospital, 28 Yeongeon-dong, Chongno-gu, Seoul 110-744, Korea
* Corresponding author.
E-mail address: sjo@snu.ac.kr

Urol Clin N Am 37 (2010) 537–546
doi:10.1016/j.ucl.2010.06.005
0094-0143/10/$ – see front matter. Published by Elsevier Inc.

Many studies have investigated whether urodynamic findings differ according to the level or the completeness of injuries. **Table 1** shows the results of a meta-analysis of 4 relevant studies on the injury level.[8–11] In summary, classification of SCI based on the level of injury gives some information, but the information seems to be insufficient for a detailed diagnosis of lower urinary tract dysfunction. Therefore, it is generally agreed that urodynamic study should be conducted to provide a precise diagnosis for each patient. In addition, little correlation between the completeness of injuries and specific urodynamic findings has been reported (**Table 2**).[9,12] The mismatch between somatic neurologic signs and urodynamic findings can be explained by the degeneration or reorganization of the neural pathway, incomplete lesions, combined lesions[9] or extension of injuries with cord fibrosis, or an aberrant healing process. The level and completeness of the injury or the existence of vascular extension usually diversifies the types of bladder dysfunction in patients with SCI. Vascular involvement makes ischemic injury extend above and below the actual level of injury.

Only a few reports have been published on TBI, especially on the correlation of urodynamic findings, because injured patients commonly have behavioral, cognitive, or communication problems. The injury to the brain itself, impairment of cognitive and behavioral function, or an associated SCI after TBI may induce voiding problems, such as incontinence. The most commonly expected urodynamic abnormality after TBI is IDC, which can be induced by the loss of cortical inhibition caused by suprapontine lesions. Coordinated relaxation of the distal sphincter during detrusor contraction is usually maintained. Asymptomatic urodynamic abnormalities were common in patients who sustained moderate or severe TBI,[13] and injuries of the frontal lobes were the most common in patients with urodynamic abnormalities.[13,14] In a high proportion of patients, frontal lobe injury could have contributed to detrusor overactivity (DO) and high incidence of urinary incontinence.[15]

The incidence of urinary retention after TBI is lower than that after cerebrovascular accident (CVA). Chua and colleagues[16] demonstrated an 8.3% retention rate after TBI, when patients were initially admitted to the rehabilitation unit, which was lower than that after CVA. The lower retention rate after TBI was likely because of the tendency toward bilateral hemispheric or subcortical involvement, which was known to be associated with IDC causing urinary incontinence or overactive bladder.[16]

Time Frame for Symptom Presentation

Bladder management in patients with SCI should vary according to time-dependent changes that occur after SCI. Within minutes of an injury, swelling of the spinal cord occurs in the spinal canal at the region of injury, which induces ischemic injury to the spinal cord tissue. In addition, bleeding may occur in the central gray matter and possibly spread to the other parts of the cord. This event causes spinal shock. Immediately after SCI, spinal shock can occur because of the absence of function below the level of cord injury. The neurophysiology of spinal shock and its recovery mechanism remain largely unknown.

Spinal shock may last from 6 to 12 weeks after complete suprasacral SCI, which can be extended to 1 or 2 years.[17] The duration of spinal shock in patients with incomplete SCI is shorter,

Table 1
Meta-analysis on the associations between injury levels and urodynamic findings in patients with SCI

	Level of Injury				
	Cervical	Thoracic	Lumbar	Sacral	*P* Value[a]
Number of Patients	259	215	137	46	
DO	65%	78%	49%	22%	<.001
DSD	63%	72%	33%	13%	<.001
DA	9%	9%	39%	70%	<.001
Normal	1%	2%	2%	9%	.002

The thoracic lesions are limited to spinal cord level T9 or above, and injuries at the T10 through T12 levels are included in lumbar lesions.[10] The combined suprasacral and sacral lesions are excluded from this analysis.[9]

Abbreviation: DO, detrusor overactivity.

[a] Pearson chi-square test.

All data are from Refs.[8–11] except data on injury at the sacral cord, which are from Refs.[8,9]

Table 2
Associations between the completeness of injury and urodynamic finding in the patients with suprasacral SCI

References	Rapidi et al[12] (n = 154)[a]			Weld and Dmochowski[9] (n = 196)[b]		
	Complete (ASIA A)	Incomplete (ASIA B)	*P* Value	Complete (ASIA A)	Incomplete (ASIA B-D)	*P* Value
DSD/DO	93%	93%	.649	100%	93%	.282
DA/DU	7%	7%		0%	3.7%	

Abbreviations: ASIA, American Spinal Injury Association classification; NS, statistically nonsignificant.
[a] Patients with cervical and thoracic lesions.
[b] The percentage is recalculated within the patients with C-L lesions. The percentage does not equal 100% because some patients with incomplete lesions manifest normal urodynamic findings.

sometimes lasting for several days.[18] Competent bladder neck and DA occur in the phase of spinal shock.[19] An electric activity can be found in the distal sphincter on electromyography. Urinary retention is therefore common, and urinary incontinence does not usually occur unless overflow incontinence exists.

As spinal shock proceeds to the recovery stage, recovery of detrusor activity is usually heralded by the recovery of skeletal muscle reflex. Therefore, the return of bulbocavernous reflex signifies recovery from spinal shock.[2] Since that time, symptoms secondary to storage difficulties start to occur between intermittent catheterization (IC). Suprasacral SCI usually causes incontinence because of IDC. As the magnitude of IDC becomes larger, postvoid residual (PVR) becomes smaller. However, the coexistence of DO with DSD results in higher voiding detrusor pressure and PVR. With sacral SCI, urinary retention may develop because of DU or DA combined with a competent distal sphincter. It should be noted that even though patients do not have severe injuries, one-third of patients with SCI need change in urological management in the absence of neurologic change. Furthermore, more than two-thirds of patients required in urological management experienced silent deterioration of bladder function on urodynamics during long-term follow-up.[20] This result emphasized the importance of regular urodynamic follow-up.

It was reported that long-term changes of bladder symptoms after TBI showed a time-dependent reduction in urinary incontinence.[16] In the acute phase, 62% of patients showed incontinence and only 9.5% of them showed a high PVR of more than 100 mL. At the time of discharge, 36.9% of them had an episode of urinary incontinence, and only 18% remained incontinent at the 6-month follow-up. A recent study also demonstrated that incontinence was the predominant symptom when the patients were admitted and that bladder impairment score improved over time.[21]

Treatment Goals and Strategies

Detailed treatment strategies should be individualized to the type of voiding dysfunction, level of injury, extent of disability, and level of care available to the patient. However, the ultimate goals of treatment in the bladder management after SCI are to preserve upper tract function with low intravesical pressure through adequate bladder drainage and to maintain urinary continence. There is no disagreement on these treatment goals among practicing urologists, although there is a lack of consensus or a standard guideline on the evaluation and management of the urinary tract.

The clinical practice guideline of the Consortium for Spinal Cord Medicine[2] reviewed various emptying or storage methods and analyzed the merits and demerits of each method when applied over long-term. This guideline commented that IC is safe and effective and that other methods may also have their own merits if applied adequately. Proposed guideline from Abrams and colleagues[22] emphasized that early clean IC (CIC) allowed easier bladder management, and patients with reflex voiding should be closely monitored on their bladder-emptying efficacy. In addition, the investigators emphasized avoidance of straining/Crede voiding.

Baseline investigation is generally performed 3 to 6 months after the initial injury, by which time spinal shock would have resolved. Baseline investigation consists of (1) general and neurologic history taking, (2) information gathering on symptoms, (3) performing neurologic examinations such as testing sacral reflexes, sacral sensation, and anal tone, (4) urinalysis, estimating serum creatinine levels, upper tract imaging, and (5) urodynamics. Nuclear renogram, voiding cystourethrography, cystoscopy, or computed tomographic scan may be needed during long-term follow-up.[17] When neurologic deficit is mild in patients with incomplete SCI, physicians sometimes omit urodynamic studies in the outpatient department. However, it is noteworthy to remember that up to half of patients with mild, incomplete injuries could develop bladder dysfunction at a later date.[20] Therefore, urodynamic studies remain valuable in the long-term follow-up of the patients with mild neurologic deficit.

Most urological centers prefer annual monitoring of upper and lower urinary tract function of patients with SCI. More-frequent follow-up is needed in the event of change in voiding pattern; development of vesicoureteral reflux (VUR), urinary tract infection (UTI), or urinary stone; change of medication; or in the presence of DSD with sustained high intravesical pressure or low compliance. Regular follow-up urodynamic studies is important to assess changes in bladder dysfunction because physiologic changes may occur even though there may be no change in overall symptoms.[23]

Treatment goals and strategies for NB related to TBI are not much different from those of NB related to CVA. In patients with TBI, the probability of recovery from incontinence is high, whereas the occurrence of DSD or low compliance, the risk factor for upper urinary tract damage, is less common.

Outcomes

Bladder emptying

The most important issue in the treatment strategy of patients with SCI is the method applied to achieve bladder emptying. IC is the most highly recommended bladder-emptying method, except in special circumstances such as inability of patients or caregiver to perform catheterization, abnormal urethral anatomy, bladder capacity less than 200 mL, and the tendency to develop autonomic dysreflexia (AD) with bladder filling.[2] Weld and Dmochowski[24] recommended CIC as the safest method of bladder emptying in patients with SCI in terms of urological complications such as infections, calculi, renal scarring, and VUR. **Table 3** compares long-term complications between IC and chronic indwelling catheterization from selected studies.[24–26] However, change in bladder management modality over time, especially bladder-emptying method, is common in patients with SCI with NB. Significant numbers of patients abandon their initial emptying methods because of inconvenience after hospital discharge.[27]

Studies suggest that the CIC method significantly improved the quality of life (QoL) in patients with SCI.[28] However, the QoL of patients with SCI was relatively reduced when compared with that of the general population.[29] This observation emphasized the importance of ongoing training to properly implement CIC and the need for psychological support in patients who rely on long-term CIC.

Reflex voiding may be used if an external containment system, such as a condom catheter, can be maintained in place. In general, when patients with SCI use triggered voiding, close urological surveillance is required because of possible coexistence of DSD. Reflex voiding is not recommended in patients with AD, high-pressure voiding, incomplete emptying, and in female patients. Valsalva or Crede voiding may

Table 3
Comparisons of long-term complications between IC and chronic indwelling catheterization in patients with SCI

Investigators	F/U (y)	Complication	IC	Chronic Indwelling Catheter	*P* Value
Weld and Dmochoski[24]	18		n = 92	n = 150	
Weld et al[25]		Patients with complications	27%	51%	<.01
		Decreased bladder compliance	26%	77%	<.01
Larsen et al[26]	12		n = 86[a]	n = 56	
		Renal-related	6 cases[b]	20 cases[b]	<.01
		Urinary tract infection	46 cases[b]	48 cases[b]	<.01
		Stones	16 cases[b]	52 cases[b]	<.01
		Urethra-related	20 cases[b]	30 cases[b]	<.01

Abbreviations: IC, intermittent catheterization; F/U, follow-up.
[a] CIC, spontaneous voiding, and external striated sphincterotomy.
[b] Some patients had more than one complications.

be considered when bladder outlet resistance is lowered and detrusor contraction is decreased simultaneously by sacral micturition center or sacral nerve root injuries. However, these methods should not be used in patients with DSD, VUR, and bladder outlet obstruction[30] and are not recommended in recent publications.[31]

Long-term indwelling catheterization is commonly used for females and individuals with high-level complete tetraplegia.[32] Shekelle and colleagues[33] reviewed 22 studies and found that CIC induced fewer UTI occurrences than the chronic indwelling catheter did. Moreover, bladder compliance is generally lower in patients using indwelling catheters than in those using other methods (see **Table 3**).[25,34,35] This difference is probably because of vesical wall fibrosis induced by inflammation and infection related to chronic indwelling catheterization.[36] For these reasons, some physicians recommend avoid long-term use of indwelling catheters, whenever possible. Additional complications related to indwelling urinary catheters are also listed in **Table 3**.

Special attention should be given to indwelling catheters and risk of bladder cancer for neurogenic bladder patients. The incidence of bladder cancer in patients with SCI is known to be 2% to 10%.[37] A recent analysis conducted by Groah and colleagues[38] on patients who used indwelling catheters for more than 12 years demonstrated that the incidence of bladder cancer is 25 times higher in patients with SCI than in the general population. However, even though the incidence of bladder cancer is higher in patients with SCI, the absolute number of individuals who develop malignancies is actually low.[2]

However, recent publications have challenged these views and suprapubic cystostomy (SPC), has been recently reported to be a safe management option for carefully selected patients if appropriate surveillance can be implemented.[39,40] Feifer and Corcos[41] reviewed 56 articles on SPC and reported that patients managed with anticholinergics, frequent urinary catheter changes and bladder washing, or volume maintenance procedures demonstrated similar morbidity to CIC. Therefore, more studies are needed on the complications of chronic indwelling of suprapubic catheters.

Striated sphincterotomy

The treatment aims of performing striated sphincterotomy are to preserve renal function, prevent sepsis, and ameliorate DSD and AD.[2] A larger series of sphincterotomy showed that significant number of patients required second operations. Recurrent UTI, DSD, and upper tract dilatation were also present in two-thirds of the patients.[42] The failures have been attributed to inadequate surgical skill, urethral strictures, and decreased detrusor contractility.[2] In addition, reasonable alternative options for refractory DSD have become available in recent years. Therefore, patients are advised to consider the efficacy and complications of different procedures before choosing an appropriate modality.

Urethral stent

Hamid and colleagues[43] investigated the long-term efficacy of urethral stent in 12 patients with DSD. Significant improvement of urodynamic parameters was found, and 7 patients continued to rely on urethral stents for more than 12 years. However, a recent study on second-generation thermoexpandable stents showed a different picture: the overall mean working life of a stent was merely 21 months.[44] Nowadays, urethral stents seem to be used only in some centers because of relatively short durability, potential complications, and difficult stent explantation for eroded or obstructing devices.

Botulinum toxin

Botulinum toxin (BTX) injection can be used for detrusor overactivity (DO) and for reducing urethral outlet resistance. BTX injection is a less-invasive alternative to sphincterotomy. BTX is effective in reducing the amount of PVR, improving maximal detrusor pressure during voiding, and managing DSD.

BTX is also effective in treating refractory neurogenic DO; however, it may have less of a therapeutic effect on patients with fibrotic changes in the bladder.[45] Most clinical studies involving BTX injections demonstrated significant improvement in clinical and urodynamic parameters without notable adverse events. Recently, the efficacy of repeated injections over a long period has been reported.[46] Although treatment with BTX has emerged as an alternative option for managing DSD and DO in recent decades, a standardized dose and an injection protocol remain to be established.

Future Developments

Sacral anterior root stimulation

Sacral posterior root rhizotomy and sacral anterior root stimulation (SARS) can be performed to manage refractory IDC and AD.[47] Electric stimulation of the sacral efferent parasympathetic nerves (S2 through S4) after dorsal rhizotomy induces bladder contraction. The result of a 7-year follow-up in 42 patients with SCI demonstrated reduced infection rate in 68% of the cohort; 54% achieved continence and 54% experienced improved social life.[48] Kutzenberger and colleagues[49] reported that

83% of patients achieved continence and most patients experienced resolution of AD. SARS has been performed for more than 30 years in a few centers and has known to be effective for micturition. However, the disadvantages of the combined rhizotomy should also be considered because of its irreversible nature.

Reinnervation of bladder by crossover nerve surgery

In 1989, Xiao and colleagues[50] suggested the feasibility of the artificial skin-central nervous system-bladder reflex pathway below the spinal cord lesion. The assumption was that the motor axons of somatic reflex arc may regenerate into autonomic preganglionic nerves, thereby reinnervating the bladder parasympathetic ganglion cells and transferring somatic reflex activity to the detrusor muscle.[51] From 1995 to 2003, the investigators performed L5 and S2/S3 ventral root microanastomoses in 15 patients with complete suprasacral SCI and found that 67% of individuals regained satisfactory bladder control during a 3-year follow-up.[52] Urodynamic study confirmed a change from DO with DSD and high detrusor pressure to nearly normal storage and synergic voiding without DSD. In addition, Xiao[51] reported that 88% of 92 patients with SCI with neurogenic DO or DA could regain bladder control 1 year after the operation. Lin and colleagues[53] reported another promising result: 75% of subjects regained satisfactory bladder control after a similar procedure in the S1 through S2/S3 region. Although this novel procedure seems promising, further studies are required to confirm the validity of its reported efficacy. Issues on tissue engineering and sacral neuromodulation are discussed in articles by Stanasel and colleagues; and Burks and colleagues elsewhere in this issue for further exploration of this topic.

VASCULAR INJURIES TO SPINAL CORD AND BRAIN

As the mortality rate associated with CVA decreases, the social cost of managing CVA survivors escalates. CVA usually occurs in elderly, and the differential diagnosis and treatment of lower urinary tract dysfunction in the patients with CVA can be confounded because of the background effects of common geriatric voiding problems, such as benign prostatic hyperplasia, overactive bladder, and stress urinary incontinence.

Spinal stroke usually makes up 1% to 2% of hospitalizations related to the vascular pathology of the nervous system.[54] Current literature indicates that aortic surgery is the dominant cause.[55] Stroke occurs most frequently at a thoracic or thoracolumbar level. Bilateral central cord is usually involved and the posterior cord is relatively spared, which means that the ischemic events predominantly affect the pyramidal and spinothalamic pathways.[56] The clinical manifestations of spinal stroke include paraplegia, which is the sensory loss below the level of the lesion. Urinary and bowel symptoms may therefore occur depending on the level of injury.

Expected Symptoms by Location of Lesion

Investigations of patients with CVA and incontinence showed the involvement of not only frontal and midbrain lesions but also parietal lesions.[57] In an animal model, a decrease of bladder capacity and the occurrence of IDC were common sequelae to cerebral infarction.[58] In the clinical setting, more than half of the patients who were symptomatic for CVA exhibited the irritative voiding symptoms and about 50% of patients with CVA complained of urinary incontinence.[59] IDC was detected in urodynamic studies in more than 80% of men who newly complained of voiding symptoms after CVA.[60] DA after CVA was, also, found in 6% of men and 19% of women complaining of urinary incontinence. However, the prevalence of incontinence showed significant time-dependent reduction.[57]

Differences in bladder dysfunction according to the location of brain lesion after CVA were investigated. **Table 4** shows the results of a meta-analysis on the associations between location of brain lesion and urodynamic findings in 133 patients with CVA.[59,61,62] A prospective study concluded that the lesions were commonly found in the frontal cortex, internal capsule, and the basal ganglia among patients with DO and that cerebellar infarction was usually related to DA.[59] However, other studies reported no such association.[61,62] Further research should be conducted to investigate whether the location of brain lesion results in different patterns of bladder dysfunction.

Differences in bladder dysfunction between ischemic and hemorrhagic lesions were also investigated. **Table 5** illustrates a meta-analysis from relevant studies.[59,63,64] Ischemic lesions were far more likely to cause DO, and hemorrhagic lesions were associated with DA.[59,64] Han and colleagues[64] suggested the possible pathophysiology of differences in urodynamics between ischemic and hemorrhagic injuries:

1. Hemorrhagic CVA usually results in a longer duration of cytotoxic edema.
2. Hemorrhagic CVA is also associated with hydrocephalus due to brain tissue displacement.

Table 4
Meta-analysis on the associations between locations of brain lesion and urodynamic findings in 133 patients with CVA

Location of the Brain Lesion	DO (%)	DA/DU (%)	Pseudo- DSD (%)	URS (%)	Normal (%)
Cerebral Cortex (n = 38)	79	18	16	26	8
Internal Capsule (n = 26)	77	15	4	50	8
Basal Ganglia (n = 24)	71	21	25	13	8
Thalamus (n = 12)	58	25	—	—	17
Combined (n = 14)	79	21	21	43	—
Pons (n = 5)	40	60	—	40	—
Cerebellum (n = 6)	—	100	—	—	—
Others (n = 8)	75	25	—	—	—

Abbreviation: URS, uninhibited relaxation of sphincter.
Data from Refs.[59,61,62]

3. Ischemic CVA usually results in cortical lesions where as hemorrhagic CVA may also involve subcortical structures.

In contrast to traumatic SCI, there is more controversy regarding urodynamic findings and level of vascular injury in the spinal cord. Siroky and colleagues[65] reported that some patients with spinal stroke at the thoracic cord sensory level showed DA. Gomelsky and colleagues[66] reported that sensory level of vascular SCI does not seem to predict urodynamic findings with consistency and that the variability of collateral arteries that feed the conus medullaris or the cauda equina from the anterior spinal cord artery may cause this discrepancy. Moreover, incomplete and patched lesions in vascular SCI could probably explain the lack of correlation.[67]

Time Frame for Symptoms

Urinary retention is commonly reported in the early period after CVA: 50% of the patients reported within 3 days[59] and 29% reported within 1 month.[68] The DA that occurs immediately after CVA may be related to immobility, aphasia, dementia, or overhydration, which can lead to bladder overdistension. However, old age itself is considered to be one of the risk factors for DA because DA is prevalent in the elderly. On the other hand, incontinence attributed to DO becomes predominant among the voiding symptoms after an early period of CVA. The incidence of incontinence was reported to be 32% to 79% in the acute stage, decreasing to 12% to 19% within 6 months after CVA.[57] The improvement of incontinence over time is very similar to that of TBI. However, older age, large lesion size, prior history of stroke or diabetes, and bowel incontinence can hinder incontinence improvement.[69]

Early development of urinary incontinence after CVA was reported to be a predictor of poor clinical outcomes, including disability and mortality.[70,71] Aphasia occurred in 74% of incontinent patients and 31% of continent patients.[72] Therefore, early development of incontinence after CVA can be helpful in distinguishing patients with poor prognoses.

Table 5
Meta-analysis on the associations between infarct types and urodynamic findings in 192 patients with CVA

Infarct Type	DO (%)	DA/DU (%)	*P* Value[a]
Ischemic type (n = 131)	69	29	<.01
Hemorrhagic type (n = 61)	36	59	

[a] Pearson chi-square test.
Data from Refs.[59,63,64]

Treatment Goals and Strategies

The most important treatment goal in patients with NB after CVA is to alleviate incontinence and irritative voiding symptoms, thereby to maintain socially acceptable dryness. Initial bladder management should be based on the urodynamic findings in symptomatic patients. Although there is no standard guideline for urodynamic evaluation, it is recommended to perform the evaluation 1 to 3 months after a stroke and then annually, considering that bladder function exhibits time-dependent changes in patients with CVA.[73] Furthermore, additional urodynamic studies are needed when patients experience changes in symptom or are under treatment.

Treatment strategies of bladder dysfunction induced by CVA are not much different from that of TBI. The presence of DO, DU, or DA and functional status, such as cognitive impairment or disability, should be evaluated first to recognize the extent of each factor affecting incontinence. Voiding dysfunction can cause difficulties in rehabilitation. As such, appropriate treatment for bladder dysfunction should be administered before discharge from the acute rehabilitation unit. When the patient first starts voiding after recovery from initial urinary retention, the frequency of performance of CIC should be determined by the amount of PVR. If incontinence is induced by DO, anticholinergics can be used, although their efficacy has not been fully validated in patients with CVA.

Outcomes

There have been a few investigations on the changes of bladder dysfunction after CVA over a long-term. It is widely accepted that post-CVA incontinence usually improves over time and it has the most negative predictability for functional recovery.[57,71,72,74] Another issue in the treatment of patients with bladder dysfunction related to CVA is the outcome of surgery such as prostatectomy or midurethral sling. Further studies are required to elucidate the efficacy of these operations in these patients.

SUMMARY

Because urological manifestations of these disease entities are highly diversified and complex, the approaches to achieve accurate diagnosis and administer proper treatment can be complicated. Complications occurring in the follow-up period are not infrequent and may result in renal deterioration. The primary treatment goal is preservation of renal function and attainment of social continence. Early identification of risk factors for a high-pressure bladder is the goal of diagnosis. Maintaining low intravesical pressure and adequate bladder emptying are central to the treatment strategy. Diagnosis and appropriate urological management of these disease entities should depend on urodynamic studies because of poor correlation between clinical symptoms or somatic neurologic signs and urodynamic findings in patients with traumatic or vascular brain injury/SCI.

REFERENCES

1. National Spinal Cord Injury Statistical Center. Facts and figures at a glance. 2009. Available at: https://www.nscisc.uab.edu/public_content/facts_figures_2009.aspx. Accessed January 14, 2010.
2. Consortium for Spinal Cord Medicine. Bladder management for adults with spinal cord injury: a clinical practice guideline for health-care providers. J Spinal Cord Med 2006;29(5):527–73.
3. Mayer SA. Head injury. In: Rowland LP, Anne MS, Joyce AM, editors. Merritt's nueology. 11th edition. Philadelphia: Lippincott Williams & Wilkins Publishing Inc; 2005. p. 483–501.
4. Tolonen A, Turkka J, Salonen O, et al. Traumatic brain injury is under-diagnosed in patients with spinal cord injury. J Rehabil Med 2007;39(8):622–6.
5. Carlsson CA. The supraspinal control of the urinary bladder. Acta Pharmacol Toxicol (Copenh) 1978;43(Suppl 2):8–12.
6. Abrams P, Cardozo L, Fall M, et al. The standardisation of terminology of lower urinary tract function: report from the Standardisation Sub-committee of the International Continence Society. Neurourol Urodyn 2002;21(2):167–78.
7. Nygaard IE, Kreder KJ. Spine update. Urological management in patients with spinal cord injuries. Spine 1996;21(1):128–32.
8. Kaplan SA, Chancellor MB, Blaivas JG. Bladder and sphincter behavior in patients with spinal cord lesions. J Urol 1991;146(1):113–7.
9. Weld KJ, Dmochowski RR. Association of level of injury and bladder behavior in patients with post-traumatic spinal cord injury. Urology 2000;55(4):490–4.
10. Wyndaele JJ. Correlation between clinical neurological data and urodynamic function in spinal cord injured patients. Spinal Cord 1997;35(4):213–6.
11. Sacomani CA, Trigo-Rocha FE, Gomes CM, et al. Effect of the trauma mechanism on the bladder-sphincteric behavior after spinal cord injury. Spinal Cord 2003;41(1):12–5.
12. Rapidi CA, Petropoulou K, Galata A, et al. Neuropathic bladder dysfunction in patients with motor complete and sensory incomplete spinal cord lesion. Spinal Cord 2008;46(10):673–8.
13. Moiyadi AV, Devi BI, Nair KP. Urinary disturbances following traumatic brain injury: clinical and urodynamic evaluation. NeuroRehabilitation 2007;22(2):93–8.
14. Oostra K, Everaert K, Van Laere M. Urinary incontinence in brain injury. Brain Inj 1996;10(6):459–64.
15. Krimchansky BZ, Sazbon L, Heller L, et al. Bladder tone in patients in post-traumatic vegetative state. Brain Inj 1999;13(11):899–903.
16. Chua K, Chuo A, Kong KH. Urinary incontinence after traumatic brain injury: incidence, outcomes and correlates. Brain Inj 2003;17(6):469–78.
17. Samson G, Cardenas DD. Neurogenic bladder in spinal cord injury. Phys Med Rehabil Clin N Am 2007;18(2):255–74.
18. Wein AJ. Lower urinary tract dysfunction in neurologic injury and disease. In: Wein AJ, Kavoussi LR, Novick AC, et al, editors. Campbell-walsh urology. 9th edition. Philadelphia: Saunders; 2007. p. 2011–45.

19. Rossier AB, Fam BA, Dibenedetto M, et al. Urodynamics in spinal shock patients. J Urol 1979;122(6):783–7.
20. Patki P, Woodhouse J, Hamid R, et al. Lower urinary tract dysfunction in ambulatory patients with incomplete spinal cord injury. J Urol 2006;175(5):1784–7.
21. Leary SM, Liu C, Cheesman AL, et al. Incontinence after brain injury: prevalence, outcome and multidisciplinary management on a neurological rehabilitation unit. Clin Rehabil 2006;20(12):1094–9.
22. Abrams P, Agarwal M, Drake M, et al. A proposed guideline for the urological management of patients with spinal cord injury. BJU Int 2008;101(8):989–94.
23. Nosseir M, Hinkel A, Pannek J. Clinical usefulness of urodynamic assessment for maintenance of bladder function in patients with spinal cord injury. Neurourol Urodyn 2007;26(2):228–33.
24. Weld KJ, Dmochowski RR. Effect of bladder management on urological complications in spinal cord injured patients. J Urol 2000;163(3):768–72.
25. Weld KJ, Graney MJ, Dmochowski RR. Differences in bladder compliance with time and associations of bladder management with compliance in spinal cord injured patients. J Urol 2000;163(4):1228–33.
26. Larsen LD, Chamberlin DA, Khonsari F, et al. Retrospective analysis of urologic complications in male patients with spinal cord injury managed with and without indwelling urinary catheters. Urology 1997;50(3):418–22.
27. Hansen RB, Biering-Sørensen F, Kristensen JK. Bladder emptying over a period of 10–45 years after a traumatic spinal cord injury. Spinal Cord 2004;42(11):631–7.
28. Vaidyananthan S, Soni BM, Brown E, et al. Effect of intermittent urethral catheterization and oxybutynin bladder instillation on urinary continence status and quality of life in a selected group of spinal cord injury patients with neuropathic bladder dysfunction. Spinal Cord 1998;36(6):409–14.
29. Oh SJ, Ku JH, Jeon HG, et al. Health-related quality of life of patients using clean intermittent catheterization for neurogenic bladder secondary to spinal cord injury. Urology 2005;65(2):306–10.
30. Giannantoni A, Scivoletto G, Di Stasi SM, et al. Clean intermittent catheterization and prevention of renal disease in spinal cord injury patients. Spinal Cord 1998;36(1):29–32.
31. Rigby D. Underactive bladder syndrome. Nurs Stand 2005;19(35):57–64.
32. Bennett CJ, Young MN, Adkins RH, et al. Comparison of bladder management complication outcomes in female spinal cord injury patients. J Urol 1995;153(5):1458–60.
33. Shekelle PG, Morton SC, Clark KA, et al. Systematic review of risk factors for urinary tract infection in adults with spinal cord dysfunction. J Spinal Cord Med 1999;22(4):258–72.
34. Cardenas DD, Mayo ME, Turner LR. Lower urinary changes over time in suprasacral spinal cord injury. Paraplegia 1995;33(6):326–9.
35. MacDiarmid SA, Arnold EP, Palmer NB, et al. Management of spinal cord injured patients by indwelling suprapubic catheterization. J Urol 1995;154(2 Pt 1):492–4.
36. Heard L, Buhrer R. How do we prevent UTI in people who perform intermittent catheterization? Rehabil Nurs 2005;30(2):44–5.
37. Bejany DE, Lockhart JL, Rhamy RK. Malignant vesical tumors following spinal cord injury. J Urol 1987;138(6):1390–2.
38. Groah SL, Weitzenkamp DA, Lammertse DP, et al. Excess risk of bladder cancer in spinal cord injury: evidence for an association between indwelling catheter use and bladder cancer. Arch Phys Med Rehabil 2002;83(3):346–51.
39. Sugimura T, Arnold E, English S, et al. Chronic suprapubic catheterization in the management of patients with spinal cord injuries: analysis of upper and lower urinary tract complications. BJU Int 2008;101(11):1396–400.
40. Mitsui T, Minami K, Furuno T, et al. Is suprapubic cystostomy an optimal urinary management in high quadriplegics? A comparative study of suprapubic cystostomy and clean intermittent catheterization. Eur Urol 2000;38(4):434–8.
41. Feifer A, Corcos J. Contemporary role of suprapubic cystostomy in treatment of neuropathic bladder dysfunction in spinal cord injured patients. Neurourol Urodyn 2008;27(6):475–9.
42. Pan D, Troy A, Rogerson J, et al. Long-term outcomes of external sphincterotomy in a spinal injured population. J Urol 2009;181(2):705–9.
43. Hamid R, Arya M, Patel HR, et al. The mesh wallstent in the treatment of detrusor external sphincter dyssynergia in men with spinal cord injury: a 12-year follow-up. BJU Int 2003;91(1):51–3.
44. Mehta SS, Tophill PR. Memokath stents for the treatment of detrusor sphincter dyssynergia (DSD) in men with spinal cord injury: the Princess Royal Spinal Injuries Unit 10-year experience. Spinal Cord 2006;44(1):1–6.
45. Schurch B, Stöhrer M, Kramer G, et al. Botulinum-A toxin for treating detrusor hyperreflexia in spinal cord injured patients: a new alternative to anticholinergic drugs? Preliminary results. J Urol 2000;164(3 Pt 1):692–7.
46. Giannantoni A, Mearini E, Del Zingaro M, et al. Six-year follow-up of botulinum toxin A intradetrusorial injections in patients with refractory neurogenic detrusor overactivity: clinical and urodynamic results. Eur Urol 2009;55(3):705–11.

47. Brindley GS, Polkey CE, Rushton DN, et al. Sacral anterior root stimulators for bladder control in paraplegia: the first 50 cases. J Neurol Neurosurg Psychiatr 1986;49(10):1104–14.
48. Vastenholt JM, Snoek GJ, Buschman HP, et al. A 7-year follow-up of sacral anterior root stimulation for bladder control in patients with a spinal cord injury: quality of life and users' experiences. Spinal Cord 2003;41(7):397–402.
49. Kutzenberger J, Domurath B, Sauerwein D. Spastic bladder and spinal cord injury: seventeen years of experience with sacral deafferentation and implantation of an anterior root stimulator. Artif Organs 2005;29(3):239–41.
50. Xiao CG, Schlossberg SM, Morgan CW, et al. A possible new reflex pathway for micturition after spinal cord injury. J Urol 1990;143:356A.
51. Xiao CG. Reinnervation for neurogenic bladder: historic review and introduction of a somatic-autonomic reflex pathway procedure for patients with spinal cord injury or spina bifida. Eur Urol 2006;49(1):22–8.
52. Xiao CG, Du MX, Dai C, et al. An artificial somatic-central nervous system-autonomic reflex pathway for controllable micturition after spinal cord injury: preliminary results in 15 patients. J Urol 2003;170(4 Pt 1):1237–41.
53. Lin H, Hou C, Zhen X, et al. Clinical study of reconstructed bladder innervation below the level of spinal cord injury to produce urination by Achilles tendon-to-bladder reflex contractions. J Neurosurg Spine 2009;10(5):452–7.
54. Nedeltchev K, Loher TJ, Stepper F, et al. Long-term outcome of acute spinal cord ischemia syndrome. Stroke 2004;35(2):560–5.
55. Salvador de la Barrera S, Barca-Buyo A, Montoto-Marqués A, et al. Spinal cord infarction: prognosis and recovery in a series of 36 patients. Spinal Cord 2001;39(10):520–5.
56. Masson C, Pruvo JP, Meder JF, et al. Spinal cord infarction: clinical and magnetic resonance imaging findings and short term outcome. J Neurol Neurosurg Psychiatr 2004;75(10):1431–5.
57. Brittain KR, Peet SM, Castleden CM. Stroke and incontinence. Stroke 1998;29(2):524–8.
58. Yokoyama O, Komatsu K, Ishiura Y, et al. Change in bladder contractility associated with bladder overactivity in rats with cerebral infarction. J Urol 1998;159(2):577–80.
59. Burney TL, Senapati M, Desai S, et al. Acute cerebrovascular accident and lower urinary tract dysfunction: a prospective correlation of the site of brain injury with urodynamic findings. J Urol 1996;156(5):1748–50.
60. Nitti VW, Adler H, Combs AJ. The role of urodynamics in the evaluation of voiding dysfunction in men after cerebrovascular accident. J Urol 1996;155(1):263–6.
61. Khan Z, Starer P, Yang WC, et al. Analysis of voiding disorders in patients with cerebrovascular accidents. Urology 1990;35(3):265–70.
62. Gupta A, Taly AB, Srivastava A, et al. Urodynamics post stroke in patients with urinary incontinence: is there correlation between bladder type and site of lesion? Ann Indian Acad Neurol 2009;12(2):104–7.
63. Ersoz M, Tunc H, Akyuz M, et al. Bladder storage and emptying disorder frequencies in hemorrhagic and ischemic stroke patients with bladder dysfunction. Cerebrovasc Dis 2005;20(5):395–9.
64. Han KS, Heo SH, Lee SJ, et al. Comparison of urodynamics between ischemic and hemorrhagic stroke patients; can we suggest the category of urinary dysfunction in patients with cerebrovascular accident according to type of stroke? Neurourol Urodyn 2009;29(3):387–90.
65. Siroky MB, Nehra A, Vlachiotis J, et al. Effect of spinal cord ischemia on vesicourethral function. J Urol 1992;148(4):1211–4.
66. Gomelsky A, Lemack GE, Weld KJ, et al. Urodynamic patterns following ischemic spinal cord events. J Urol 2003;170(1):122–5.
67. Luján Marco S, García Fadrique G, Ramírez Backhaus M, et al. Urological findings in spinal cord ischemia. Actas Urol Esp 2008;32(9):926–30.
68. Kolominsky-Rabas PL, Hilz MJ, Neundoerfer B, et al. Impact of urinary incontinence after stroke: results from a prospective population-based stroke register. Neurourol Urodyn 2003;22(4):322–7.
69. Patel M, Coshall C, Lawrence E, et al. Recovery from poststroke urinary incontinence: associated factors and impact on outcome. J Am Geriatr Soc 2001;49(9):1229–33.
70. Taub NA, Wolfe CD, Richardson E, et al. Predicting the disability of first-time stroke sufferers at 1 year. 12-month follow-up of a population-based cohort in southeast England. Stroke 1994;25(2):352–7.
71. Nakayama H, Jørgensen HS, Pedersen PM, et al. Prevalence and risk factors of incontinence after stroke. The Copenhagen Stroke Study. Stroke 1997;28(1):58–62.
72. Gelber DA, Good DC, Laven LJ, et al. Causes of urinary incontinence after acute hemispheric stroke. Stroke 1993;24(3):378–82.
73. Burney TL, Senapati M, Desai S, et al. Effects of cerebrovascular accident on micturition. Urol Clin North Am 1996;23(3):483–90.
74. Turhan N, Atalay A, Atabek HK. Significance of post-stroke urinary incontinence as a negative predictor of functional recovery on the basis of aging. J Am Geriatr Soc 2006;54(6):1022–3.

Contemporary Management of the Neurogenic Bladder for Multiple Sclerosis Patients

John T. Stoffel, MD

KEYWORDS

- Urinary bladder • Neurogenic • Multiple sclerosis
- Therapeutics

EPIDEMIOLOGY OF MULTIPLE SCLEROSIS

Multiple sclerosis (MS) is the most common neuroinflammatory disease of the central nervous system (CNS), and is characterized by plaques of demyelination in CNS white matter. The disease affects approximately 85 cases per 100,000 people[1] and is more prevalent in northern than southern latitudes. The initial onset of neurologic symptoms typically occurs between ages 20 and 50 years, and presentation at an age older than 40 may be associated with a greater risk of progressive disability.[2,3] Women are 2 to 4 times more commonly affected than men.[4] Although researchers have cited the Epstein-Barr virus, ultraviolet radiation, tobacco, vitamin D deficiency, and smoked meat with nitrites as potential environmental risk factors for developing MS,[4,5] familial clustering and twin studies suggest risk is more related to a complex interaction between genetically susceptible patients and their specific environments.[6,7]

CLASSIFICATION

Clinically, MS presents as acute neurologic compromise, and most patients cite symptoms of numbness, decreased of motor strength, and loss of coordination and/or vision. MS can be diagnosed by the McDonald Criteria, which require magnetic resonance imaging (MRI) findings to correlate with 2 neurologic clinical manifestations, separated by time and recovery. A spinal tap showing oligodonal bands also supports the diagnosis when no recovery has occurred.[8] Disability is commonly reported in the literature through the Extended Disability Symptom Score (EDSS), which measures disease impact on pyramidal (voluntary), brainstem, visual, cerebral (memory), cerebellar, sensory, and bowel/bladder systems. A single score is given, which ranges from 1 (minimal impact) to 10 (death from disease). Patients with scores higher than 6.5 require constant bilateral assistance to walk 20 m without resting and have impact on 2 systems.[9] The severity of urinary symptoms appears to be associated with EDSS scores and usually correlates with pyramidal symptom severity.[10]

MS can be roughly categorized into 3 different disease progressions[11]:

Relapsing/Remitting: Eighty percent of MS patients will experience symptoms followed by complete or partial resolution after 2 days to 6 weeks. There is no progression of disease between episodes. The initial relapse rate is approximately 0.3 episodes per year, but frequency decreases as time progresses.

Secondary Progressive: Fifty percent of relapsing/remitting patients will develop progressive neurologic decline, particularly

Department of Urology, Lahey Clinic, 41 Mall Road, Burlington, MA 01805, USA
E-mail address: john_t_stoffel@lahey.org

Urol Clin N Am 37 (2010) 547–557
doi:10.1016/j.ucl.2010.06.003
0094-0143/10/$ – see front matter

in the lower extremities. Secondary Progressive MS typically occurs more than 10 years after initial diagnosis and is characterized by less recovery from symptomatic episodes.

Primary Progressive: Ten percent of patients will experience continuous neurologic degradation after initial presentation, characterized by no remission.

MS AND BLADDER PHYSIOLOGY

Impact of Lesion Location

Imaging and anatomic studies suggest that patients with MS lesions located in specific CNS regions are more likely to display prominent urinary symptoms. In general, lesion volume modestly correlates with symptom progression within the first 5 years.[12] Charil and colleagues[13] studied 452 MRI scans from relapsing and remitting MS patients, and found patients with lesions in the medial frontal lobes, cerebellum, insula, dorsal midbrain, and pons scored significantly lower on urinary-specific quality of life assessments. Likewise, other studies have found a strong association on MRI between midbrain lesions and loss of urinary control.[14,15] Patients with cerebellar or specific frontal lobe lesions may display urinary incontinence or urinary retention due to loss of cognitive function or awareness of bladder volumes.[16,17] Spinal plaques affecting the corticospinal tracts are also common, and are responsible for symptom progression measured by the EDSS.[18] Up to 80% of MS patients will have cervical spinal cord involvement[19] and are likely to display some urinary hesitancy and retention.[20]

With the exception of detrusor-external dyssynergia (DSD), there is conflicting evidence regarding lesion location and specific, reproducible urodynamic findings. Kim evaluated 90 patients with symptomatic MS (EDSS scores not reported) and found no clear relationship between urodynamic findings, MRI lesion location, International Prostate Symptom Scores, and lesion size.[21] Other studies reported some associations between high-volume cortical lesions and detrusor overactivity,[22] pontine lesions and detrusor areflexia,[23] and pontine to conus medullaris lesions and ice water–induced detrusor contractions.[24] Sacral cord lesions are less common in MS but can be associated with detrusor hypocontractility and atony on urodynamic study.[17] Detrusor-sphincter dyssynergia appears to have a strong correlation with MS lesions in the cervical spinal cord.[22,23,25] A strong relationship between DSD and cervical spinal cord lesions or injuries has also been described in spinal cord injury pathologies.[26]

Impact of Disease Process

MS likely causes clinical symptoms, including urinary symptoms, through demyelization and axonal degradation.[11,27] Demyelination is thought to develop before degradation. Using experimental autoimmune encephalomyelitis animal models, research suggests that CD4+ and CD8+ T cells along with macrophages induce and then maintain an inflammatory reaction against the axonal myelin sheath, which ultimately results in demyelination.[11] Autoimmune antibodies from B calls may also play a role in maintaining inflammation along the axon.[28] Axonal degradation may occur over time as the axon becomes more vulnerable to stress and degrades due to inhibition of remyelination, exposure of an increased number of Na^+ channels, and decreased adenosine triphosphate production in the demyelinated area.[11,29,30] Although there is a clear relationship between plaque development and clinical symptoms, axonal degradation may be more strongly associated with progression of symptoms than previously appreciated.

MS CNS lesions may also exert a local effect on the bladder function. It is known that any CNS lesion can cause previously silent unmyelinated C fibers in the bladder to become increasingly mechanosensitive to detrusor wall stretching.[31] Radziszewski and colleagues[32] performed urodynamics and trigonal bladder biopsies from 18 symptomatic MS patients, and found a greater density of substance P and calcitonin gene related peptide–sensitive unmyelinated C fibers in patients with detrusor overactivity. Findings such as these suggest that biopsies measuring C-fiber neuronal density may be used in the future to gauge a patient's potential response to intravesical treatments. Other changes in bladder structure may also occur in the setting of MS, such as alterations in the ultrastructure of the bladder lamina propria[33] and increased number of Schwann cells.[34] The clinical impact of these findings is unclear, and more research is needed to correlate pathology with clinical symptoms.

Presentation of Urinary Symptoms

In the North American Research Committee on Multiple Sclerosis (NARCOMS) cross-sectional survey of 9700 MS patients, 65% reported at least moderate to severe urinary symptoms.[35] Urinary urgency is usually the most prevalent reported symptom for MS patients. Compared with an unaffected population in a cross-sectional study of 12,570 Canadian women, patients with multiple sclerosis were 7.6 times more likely to report bother from overactive bladder symptoms.[36] In some studies, up to 21% to 50% of patients experience frequent episodes of urinary incontinence in addition to hesitancy and 25% of patients report frank urinary retention.[35,37,38] Phadke's review[3] of MS epidemiology suggests that 0% to 14% of MS patients will report urinary complaints as the initial MS symptom and mean time to onset of symptomatic urinary dysfunction for most MS patient ranges between 6[39] and 8 years[40] after initial diagnosis. However, changes in urinary symptoms have been noted as early as 2 years after initial diagnosis are usually associated with an increasing postvoid residual (PVR) and a worse disease course.[3,41]

CLINICAL EVALUATIONS

Urodynamics

Urinary symptom type does not always predict urodynamic findings because different voiding dysfunction pathologies can present with the same common urinary complaint. In a prospective study of 212 MS patients by Koldewijn and colleagues,[10] 27% complained of obstructive/retention urinary symptoms. When examined with urodynamic tests, 8% of the sample had detrusor hypoactivity, 13% had DSD, and 5% had other unspecified bladder outlet obstruction. Other investigators have also commented on the low correlation between urinary symptoms and urodynamic findings for MS patients.[42,43] Furthermore, 70% of MS patients presented with combined symptoms of obstruction and incontinence in one study,[44] suggesting that multiple voiding dysfunction patterns can coexist.

MS patients at the author's institution undergo urodynamic testing for symptoms of refractory urinary incontinence, obstruction/hesitancy, urinary retention, and elevated PVR greater than 150. All urodynamic studies for MS patients should use standardized approved urodynamics practice recommendations from the International Continence Society.[45] Electromyography and/or fluoroscopy are needed to diagnose DSD during the studies, but there is no consensus on the best technique for identifying this pathology.[20,46,47] The author relies on electromyography (EMG) to assess DSD and has found fluoroscopy to be helpful in identifying DSD, bladder diverticuli, and vesicoureteral reflux.

There are multiple small descriptive studies reporting on urodynamic findings in MS patients. Litwiller and colleagues[17] performed a meta-analysis on urodynamic data from 22 studies, comprising of 1882 MS patients, and found detrusor overactivity (then called hyperreflexia) in 62% of the total sample, DSD in 25%, hyporeflexia in 20%, and no findings in 10%. There are data suggesting that MS patients with neurogenic detrusor overactivity will demonstrate greater amplitude of detrusor contraction compared with idiopathic detrusor overactivity.[48] Of note, MS women with DSD did not display higher voiding pressures in a subsequent study.[49] New urodynamic findings can present or old findings change as the disease progresses. Ciancio and colleagues[50] followed 14 MS patients over a mean 42-month follow-up, and found 5 patients with lower bladder compliance and 6 with new voiding pathologies. Given the multiple and changing urodynamic findings in MS patients, the author believes that patients can benefit from serial urodynamic testing as the disease progresses.

Urinary Tract Infections

Urinary tract infections (UTI) are also prevalent in the MS population, and patients with DSD may be at particular risk for pyelonephritis.[51] Evidence suggests that systemic bacteria infections may exacerbate the autoimmune response in MS.[52,53] The frequency at which an MS patient experiences UTI may also increase the risk of symptom progression.[54,55] Risk factors for UTI have not been completely identified, although an elevated PVR and DSD may be potential variables.[40,51] More research is needed to identify other potential risk factors unique to the MS population. Expert opinion suggests that all MS patients with symptomatic, recurrent UTIs be evaluated with a PVR and upper tract imaging studies.[56] At the author's institution, urodynamics is also performed to evaluate dysfunction voiding physiology as a risk factor.

Upper Tract Changes

There is considerable controversy surrounding MS and risk of upper urinary tract degeneration. The reported prevalence of upper tract changes in the MS population has ranged widely from 0.9% to 17%.[10,57–59] de Sèze and colleagues[40] compiled data from 11 studies consisting of 1200 MS patients and found a rising incidence of upper tract complications over time for patients symptomatic with MS. These data suggested that upper tract changes were most likely to occur after 6 to 8 years with disease. Time with disease, increased patient age, and pyramidal symptoms have also been associated with an increased risk for upper tract changes in some studies,[57,60] but others do not associate upper tract changes with any risk factors.[58,59] Care should be applied when extrapolating data from these studies because patients in each cohort could represent different patient populations, access to care, and different MS treatment regimens.

Cancer

Bahmanyar and colleagues[61] assessed cancer risk in 20,276 MS patients over 35 years of follow-up and found an increased risk for developing urinary organ cancer, excluding kidney, prostate (hazard ratio 1.27, 95% confidence interval 1.05–1.53). The cause of this is unclear, but it may represent surveillance bias. In addition, MS patients treated with cyclophosphamide may be at increased risk for bladder cancer.[62]

TREATMENT

In a disease marked by relatively poor control of symptoms, urinary complaints are a point of intervention that can be addressed and improved for a large number of MS patients. Maintaining adequate urinary control may also have additional benefits on sexual health and mental health, particularly in MS patients with increasing disability.[41] Consequently, a plan of increasing intervention can be employed to address both safety- and urinary-specific quality of life for these complex patients. The treatment plan used at the author's institution is presented in **Fig. 1**. Additional algorithms have also been published.[40,56,63]

Behavioral Therapy

Behavioral therapy, including interventions such as pelvic floor muscle training (PFMT) and fluid management, has been an effective treatment strategy for women with idiopathic overactive bladder symptoms.[64] Because many MS patients have pelvic floor muscle spasms in addition to voiding dysfunction,[65] PFMT therapies, in theory, can yield some symptomatic improvements. However, there are few studies examining the efficacy of behavioral therapy for neurogenic detrusor overactivity related to MS. De Ridder and colleagues[66] demonstrated improvement in mean functional bladder capacity (178 mL to 205 mL) and reduction in mean number of urinary frequency episodes (12.7 to 9.1) after 1 month of PFMT. Combining behavioral therapy modalities

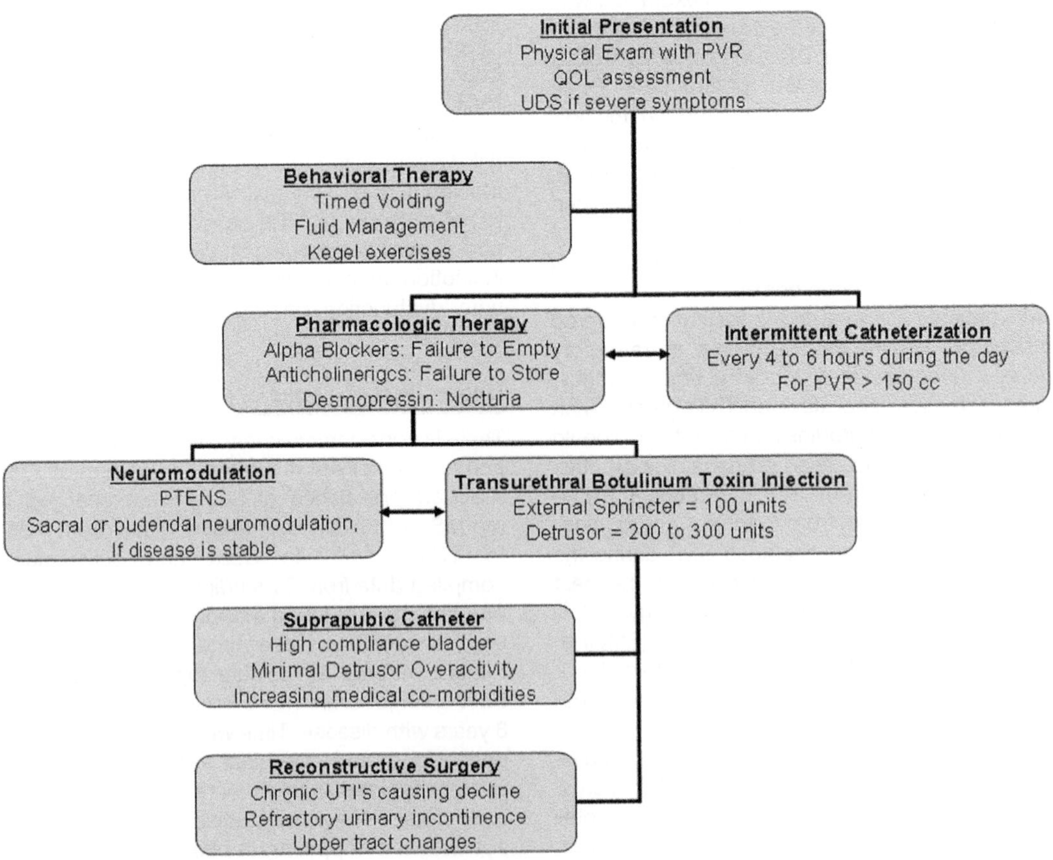

Fig. 1. Treatment options for MS-related urinary symptoms. DSD, detrusor-sphincter dyssynergia; PTENS, percutaneous electrical nerve stimulation; PVR, postvoid residual; QOL, quality of life; UDS, urodynamic studies; UTI, urinary tract infection.

may also offer benefit for MS patients. McClurg and colleagues[67] randomized 30 women with MS into treatment groups of PFMT, PFMT + EMG biofeedback, and PFMT + EMG biofeedback + neuromuscular stimulation, and found improved efficacy in reducing the number of leaking episodes (P = .014) and in volume leaked (P = .0001) when all 3 modalities were used compared with PFMT alone or PFMT + EMG. A larger double-blinded study by the same group noted an 85% reduction of urinary incontinence episodes with neuromuscular stimulation + EMG + PFMT, compared with 47% reduction in the PFMT + EMG + placebo group.[68]

Pharmacologic Therapy

Oral pharmacologic therapy in the MS population targets 3 prevalent urinary symptoms: urgency/urge incontinence, urinary retention, and nocturia.

Anticholinergics

Although anticholinergic medications are recommend to treat urge/urge incontinence in multiple sclerosis,[69] there are few studies examining efficacy. Fader and colleagues[70] compared intravesical atropine to oxybutynin immediate release and found a small difference in posttreatment bladder capacity (55 mL improvement with oxybutynin vs 79 mL with atropine) but no difference in incidence of incontinence events. Other studies have also demonstrated symptom improvement with increasing anticholinergic medication dosage,[71] or using anticholinergics to convert detrusor overactivity to detrusor hypocontractility.[43] However, Nicholas and colleagues[72] performed an analysis on all current literature regarding anticholinergic therapy for MS-related incontinence and found only 5 usable studies, none of which included placebos or long-acting anticholinergic medications. No conclusions suggesting benefit from anticholinergic usage could be drawn from the analysis. In addition to the lack of outcome studies, physicians are likely undertreating urgency/urge incontinence in the MS population. According to the NARCOM survey, only 43% of patients with significant urinary urgency had seen a urologist and only 51% were treated with an anticholinergic.[35] Alternative pharmacologic agents, such as cannabis, have demonstrated some efficacy in reducing MS-related urinary incontinence,[73] but use of this medication is only investigational at this point in time.

α-Blockers

There is also little information regarding pharmacologic treatment of MS-related urinary retention. O'Riordan and colleagues[74] noted a 41% improvement in flow rate and a 26% reduction of PVR with MS patients treated with an α-blocker for 4 weeks. Stankovich and colleagues[75] noted a 54% decrease in International Prostate Symptom Score for 28 MS patients (20 female) with DSD who were treated with tamsulosin, 0.4 mg for 2 months. Additional studies of mixed DSD pathologies, including MS, also found tamsulosin to be effective in treating obstructive symptoms.[76]

Desmopressin

By contrast, there are many studies investigating the efficacy of desmopressin, 20 μg, for MS-related nocturia. While on desmopressin, MS patients experienced a decrease in nocturia by mean 0.5 to 1.5 episodes per night and an increase of uninterrupted sleep by mean 2 hours.[77–79] A high bladder capacity and compliance may predict better outcomes for desmopressin in MS patients.[78] Reduction in urinary frequency is limited to the first 6 to 8 hours after delivery. Urine sodium and maximal urinary daily output remained relatively stable in a meta-analysis of MS patients on desmopressin.[79]

Catheterization

MS patients may require some assistance in bladder emptying because of DSD, detrusor atony, and/or reduced physical mobility. In the NARCOMS survey, 37% of MS patients reported using catheter assistance for bladder emptying. Catheter usage correlated with advance disease.[35] Although the PVR volume which places patients at most risk for urinary pathologies is not known, the United Kingdom consensus on management for multiple sclerosis urinary symptoms recommends teaching clean intermittent catheterization (CIC) to patients with PVRs greater than 100 mL.[63] In most CIC treatment plans, patients catheterize according to a set time schedule, ranging from every 3 to 6 hours. CIC can be easily taught to most MS patients, and at least one study reported successful CIC education for 87% of MS patients. However, more instruction was needed for patients with cognitive decline and higher EDSS.[80] Fakas and colleagues[81] examined the risk of UTIs for MS patients on CIC, and found that while 90% of these patients developed bacteriuria, only 14% developed symptomatic urinary tract infections. In general, CIC seems to be a safe, well-tolerated management strategy for the symptomatic MS patient.

However, controversy surrounds the use of indwelling urinary catheters for refractory MS urinary symptoms. Although studies have demonstrated severe urethral damage and erosion from long-term urethral catheterization in MS patients,[82,83] the true incidence of urethral and bladder complications from urethral catheters is not known for the MS population. If an indwelling catheter is indicated, the United Kingdom consensus statement recommends offering a suprapubic instead of a urethral catheter.[63] Although commonly used, long-term complications of suprapubic catheterization have not been reported for the MS population regarding patient satisfaction, rate of UTI, loss of bladder compliance, and risk of bladder cancer.

Intravesical Agents/Botulinum Toxin

Intravesical agents have been used to treat MS-related urinary urgency and incontinence. Several trials of mixed multiple sclerosis and spinal cord injury patients have found intravesical installations of capsaicin or resiniferatoxin superior to placebo in reducing neurogenic urinary urgency/frequency.[84–86] When comparing these vanilloid agents, resiniferatoxin treatments resulted in fewer incontinent episodes per day (60% improvement with capsaicin, 94% improvement with resiniferatoxin) and capsaicin treatments were associated with more short-term pubic pain during installation.[87] However, a meta-analysis did not yield a consistent treatment effect for vanilloid agents.[88] Given the questionable efficacy of anticholinergics in treating MS-related urgency/incontinence, more research is needed to develop an efficacious, easy to use, intravesical agent for the symptomatic MS patient.

Botulinum toxin A injections represent a significant advancement in treatment options for neurogenic voiding dysfunction. Although there are no evidence-based guidelines suggesting optimal injection location or dose, 10 units/mL injections usually are spaced across the posterior detrusor and the trigone is spared to minimize the risk of vesicoureteral reflux.[69] There are multiple trials that suggest intradetrusor botulinum toxin injections can improve cystometric capacity by 50% to 300%, improve time to first desire by 50%, and reduce the number of incontinence episodes by 40% to 77%.[89–97] Botulinum toxin has also been used to decrease urethral leakage in the setting of an indwelling urinary catheter.[98] In contrast to the spinal cord injury literature, botulinum toxin injections into the external sphincter did not demonstrate improvement in PVR in a recent placebo-controlled trial,[96] but smaller observational trials have suggested efficacy (**Table 1**). In general, toxin efficacy is limited in duration, and most studies suggest benefits begin to wane after 6 months.[89–97] Botulinum toxin–specific a ntibodies have also been detected

Table 1
Botulinum toxin therapy for multiple sclerosis voiding dysfunction

Study	N (% MS)	Dosage	Outcome	Comments
Werfer (2009)[89]	214 (5)	290	58% reduction in UTI incidence	Cost $830 (617 euro)/year per patient
Ehren (2007)[90]	31 (20)	500	Improvement in capacity, compared to placebo	All patients on tolteridine Dyport used
Gamé (2007)[91]	30 (50)	300	53% improvement in time to 1st desire	Reduction in UTI incidence, pediatric study
Kalsi (2007)[92]	43 (100)	300	300% increase in capacity 45% decrease frequency 77% incontinence episodes	98% performed CIC after
Schurch (2007)[93]	59 (10)	200–300	−1.1 incontinence/day episode reduction	Significant at 24 weeks
Schulte-Baukloh (2006)[94]	16 (100)	300	58–77% improvement in max capacity 38–64% pad use reduction	Injection to both external sphincter and detrusor
Popat (2005)[95]	44 (66)	300	53% improvement in max capacity, incontinence	
Gallen (2005)[96]	86 (100)	100	No change in PVR	Injection into external sphincter only for DSD
Smith (2005)[97]	110 (43)	100–300	PVR reduction (sphincter) 40% incontinence reduction (bladder injection)	Injection into both bladder or urethra

after injections and may be a source of treatment failure over time.[99] At present, botulinum toxin is not approved by the US Food and Drug Administration for use in the bladder. Consequently, treating physicians should obtain detailed informed consent from patients and follow institution guidelines for off-label medication usage.

Neuromodulation

Given the likely neurogenic source of voiding dysfunction in MS patients, neuromodulation offers great potential for alleviating symptoms. Sacral nerve stimulation has been attempted for both urinary retention and detrusor overactivity in MS patients. In one series of 14 patients with a mean EDSS of 4, PVRs have decreased from a mean 308 to 50 mL over a mean 4-year follow-up.[100] Another study comprising 33 patients with MS and other neurogenic causes of voiding dysfunction noted a 58% reduction of CIC episodes per 24 hours after neuromodulation.[101] Similar improvement in urinary urgency and incontinence episodes have been reported in other small neuromodulation trials containing some MS patients.[101,102]

However, an implantable sacral nerve stimulator precludes further MRI evaluations. Consequently, alternative nonimplantable neuromodulation modalities have been investigated for use in MS patients. Percutaneous dorsal penile/clitoral nerve stimulation resulted in a mean 95% increase in bladder capacity[103] and posterior tibial nerve stimulation improved bladder capacity by 67%[104] in trials of 10 and 27 MS patients, respectively. However, additional posterior tibial and sacral dermatome stimulation trials did not demonstrate urodynamic improvements.[105,106] At present, sacral nerve stimulation appears to be more effective than posterior tibial or dorsal penile/clitoral stimulation. Pudendal nerve stimulation offers some theoretical benefits over sacral nerve stimulation, but no data are yet available on outcomes in MS patients.

Urinary Diversion/Reconstruction

Surgical intervention for MS-related voiding dysfunction can be performed for select patients. Indications include refractory urinary incontinence causing skin complications, chronic UTIs related to incomplete urinary drainage or chronic catheterization, catheter-associated erosions, and renal compromise from low bladder compliance or reflux. In general, most patients considering surgical intervention have secondary progressive/primary progressive disease, have failed nonsurgical treatment modalities, and have increasing EDSS. Before committing to urinary diversion/reconstruction, a thorough discussion regarding current rate of disease progression, expectations, risks, and benefits needs to occur between neurologist, urologist, patient, and family.

There are few dedicated surgical series on surgical outcomes and complications for MS patients. End points are rarely standardized and follow-up is generally short. Regarding endoscopic treatment of DSD for MS patients, Gamé and colleagues[107] tested 147 patients, including 24 with MS, and reported that 71% progressed on to a permanent urethral wall stent implantation. Little additional information regarding efficacy and quality of life is available for this modality or for transurethral sphincterotomy.

Some MS patients with low bladder capacity/compliance may benefit from augmentation cystoplasty and/or continent catheterizable stomas. Auotaugmentation has been reported as an option for improving low bladder compliance,[108] and Zachoval and colleagues[109] noted enterocystoplasty to have good efficacy for treating urinary symptoms in a cohort of 9 symptomatic MS patients (EDSS = 4.1). The author has performed enterocystoplasty in 5 MS patients and has noted improvement in urethral continence and reduction of UTIs after surgery. However, long-term outcomes of enterocystoplasty and impact on disease progression is not known.

At the author's institution, most MS patients needing surgical intervention will require an incontinent urinary diversion due patient inability to catheterize or maintain mobility. Ileovesicostomy procedures have improved urinary symptoms in several mixed pathology series, although complications regarding wound infections, stones, and continued urinary incontinence have been considerable.[110–112] The author's group has reported good short-term efficacy using a robotic-assisted ileovesicostomy procedure for MS patients that may offer a decreased risk of wound infections.[113] There is also a small series reporting ileal loop as a viable urinary diversion for treating MS patients with refractory urinary symptoms.[114] At his institution, the author has performed 19 urinary diversions for MS patients (Mean EDSS = 6.5), including 15 ileovesicostomy and 4 ileal loop procedures, found that surgical intervention decreased incidence of UTIs, improved urethral continence, and preserved upper tract safety. Follow-up from this series is currently too short to assess the impact of intervention on disease progression.

SUMMARY

Patients with MS sclerosis have a high incidence of urinary complaints. Urologists educated in MS pathophysiology and contemporary treatment options can greatly improve safety and quality of life for these symptomatic patients.

REFERENCES

1. Noonan CW, Kathman SJ, White MC. Prevalence estimates for MS in the United States and evidence of an increasing trend for women. Neurology 2002;58:136–8.
2. Detels R, Clark VA, Valdiviezo NL, et al. Factors associated with a rapid course of multiple sclerosis. Arch Neurol 1982;39:337–41.
3. Phadke JG. Clinical aspects of multiple sclerosis in North-East Scotland with particular reference to course and prognosis. Brain 1990;113:1597–628.
4. Noonan CW, Williamson DM, Henry JP, et al. The prevalence of multiple sclerosis in 3 US communities. Prev Chronic Dis 2010;7:A12.
5. Lauer K. Environmental risk factors in multiple sclerosis. Expert Rev Neurother 2010;10:421–40.
6. Milo R, Kahana E. Multiple sclerosis: geoepidemiology, genetics and the environment. Autoimmun Rev 2010;9:A387–94.
7. Hemminki K, Li X, Sundquist J, et al. Risk for multiple sclerosis in relatives and spouses of patients diagnosed with autoimmune and related conditions. Neurogenetics 2009;10:5–11.
8. McDonald WI, Compston A, Edan G, et al. Recommended diagnostic criteria for multiple sclerosis: guidelines from the international panel on the diagnosis of multiple sclerosis. Ann Neurol 2001;50(1):121–7.
9. Gaspari M, Roveda G, Scandellari C, et al. An expert system for the evaluation of EDSS in multiple sclerosis. Artif Intell Med 2002;25:187–210.
10. Koldewijn EL, Hommes OR, Lemmens AJG, et al. Relationship between lower urinary tract abnormalities and disease-related parameters in multiple sclerosis. J Urol 1995;154:169–73.
11. Siffrin V, Vogt J, Radbruch H, et al. Multiple sclerosis—candidate mechanisms underlying CNS atrophy. Trends Neurosci 2010;33:202–10.
12. Brex PA, Ciccarelli O, O'Riordan JI, et al. A longitudinal study of abnormalities on MRI and disability from multiple sclerosis. N Engl J Med 2002;346:158–64.
13. Charil A, Zijdenbos AP, Taylor J, et al. Statistical mapping analysis of lesion location and neurological disability in multiple sclerosis: application to 452 patient data sets. Neuroimage 2003;19:532–44.
14. Grasso MG, Pozzilli C, Anzini A, et al. Relationship between bladder dysfunction and brain MRI in multiple sclerosis. Funct Neurol 1991;6:289–92.
15. Pozzilli C, Grasso MG, Bastianello S, et al. Structural brain correlates of neurologic abnormalities in multiple sclerosis. Eur Neurol 1992;32:228–30.
16. Abou Zeid NE, Weinshenker BG, Keegan BM. Gait apraxia in multiple sclerosis. Can J Neurol Sci 2009;36:562–5.
17. Litwiller SE, Frohman EM, Zimmern PE. Multiple sclerosis and the urologist. J Urol 1999;161:743–57.
18. Tartaglino LM, Friedman DP, Flander AE, et al. Multiple sclerosis and the spinal cord: MR appearance and correlation with clinical parameters. Radiology 1995;195:725–32.
19. Oppenheimer DR. The cervical cord in multiple sclerosis. Neuropathol Appl Neurobiol 1978;4:151–62.
20. McGuire EJ, Savastano JA. Urodynamic findings and long-term outcome management of patients with multiple sclerosis-induced lower urinary tract dysfunction. J Urol 1984;132:713–5.
21. Kim YH, Goodman C, Omessi E, et al. The correlation of urodynamic findings with cranial magnetic resonance imaging findings in multiple sclerosis. J Urol 1998;159:972–6.
22. Ukkonen M, Elovaara I, Dastidar P, et al. Urodynamic findings in primary progressive multiple sclerosis are associated with increased volumes of plaques and atrophy in the central nervous system. Acta Neurol Scand 2004;109:100–5.
23. Araki I, Matsui M, Ozawa K, et al. Relationship of bladder dysfunction to lesion site in multiple sclerosis. J Urol 2003;169:1384–7.
24. Ismael SS, Epstein T, Bayle B, et al. Bladder cooling reflex in patients with multiple sclerosis. J Urol 2000;164:1280–4.
25. Hinson JL, Boone TB. Urodynamics and multiple sclerosis. Urol Clin North Am 1996;23:475–81.
26. Kaplan SA, Chancellor MB, Blaivas JG. Bladder and sphincter behavior in patients with spinal cord lesions. J Urol 1991;146:113–7.
27. Dutta R, Trapp BD. Pathogenesis of axonal and neuronal damage in multiple sclerosis. Neurology 2007;68:S22–31 [discussion: S43–54].
28. Bartos A, Fialová L, Soukupová J, et al. Elevated intrathecal antibodies against the medium neurofilament subunit in multiple sclerosis. J Neurol 2007;254:20–5.
29. Mahad DJ, Ziabreva I, Campbell G, et al. Mitochondrial changes within axons in multiple sclerosis. Brain 2009;132:1161–74.
30. Trapp BD, Stys PK. Virtual hypoxia and chronic necrosis of demyelinated axons in multiple sclerosis. Lancet Neurol 2009;8:280–91.
31. de Groat WC, Yoshimura N. Changes in afferent activity after spinal cord injury. Neurourol Urodyn 2010;29:63–76.
32. Radziszewski P, Crayton R, Zaborski J, et al. Multiple sclerosis produces significant changes in urinary bladder innervation which are partially reflected in the lower urinary tract functional

status-sensory nerve fibers role in detrusor overactivity. Mult Scler 2009;15:860–8.
33. Wiseman OJ, Brady CM, Hussain IF, et al. The ultrastructure of bladder lamina propria nerves in healthy subjects and patients with detrusor hyperreflexia. J Urol 2002;168:2040–5.
34. Van Poppel H, Stessens R, Lazarides M, et al. Neuropathological examination of the alterations of the intrinsic innervation in multiple sclerosis cystopathy. Urol Int 1989;44:321–6.
35. Mahajan ST, Patel PB, Marrie RA. Under treatment of overactive bladder symptoms in patients with multiple sclerosis: an ancillary analysis of the NARCOMS Patient Registry. J Urol 2010;183:1432–7.
36. McGrother CW, Donaldson MM, Hayward T, et al. Urinary storage symptoms and comorbidities: a prospective population cohort study in middle-aged and older women. Age Ageing 2006;35:16–24.
37. Nakipoglu GF, Kaya AZ, Orhan G, et al. Urinary dysfunction in multiple sclerosis. J Clin Neurosci 2009;16:1321–4.
38. Khan F, Pallant JF, Shea TL, et al. Multiple sclerosis: prevalence and factors impacting bladder and bowel function in an Australian community cohort. Disabil Rehabil 2009;31:1567–76.
39. Betts CD, D'Mellow MT, Fowler CJ. Urinary symptoms and neurologic features of bladder dysfunction in multiple sclerosis. J Neurol Neurosurg Psychiatry 1993;56:245–50.
40. de Sèze M, Ruffion A, Denys P, et al. The neurogenic bladder in multiple sclerosis: review of the literature and proposal of management guidelines. Mult Scler 2007;13:915–28.
41. Nortvedt MW, Riise T, Frugård J, et al. Prevalence of bladder, bowel and sexual problems among multiple sclerosis patients 2 to 5 years after diagnosis. Mult Scler 2007;13:106–12.
42. Blaivas JG. Management of bladder dysfunction in multiple sclerosis. Neurology 1980;30:12–8.
43. Sirls LT, Zimmern PE, Leach GE. Role of limited evaluation and aggressive medical management in multiple sclerosis: a review of 113 patients. J Urol 1994;151:946–50.
44. Onal B, Siva A, Buldu I, et al. Voiding dysfunction due to multiple sclerosis: a large scale retrospective analysis. Int Braz J Urol 2009;35:326–33.
45. Schäfer W, Abrams P, Liao L, et al. Good urodynamic practices: uroflowmetry, filling cystometry, and pressure-flow studies. Neurourol Urodyn 2002;21:261–74.
46. Dibenedetto M, Yalla SV. Electrodiagnosis of striated urethral sphincter dysfunction. J Urol 1979;122:361–5.
47. Koyanagi T, Takamatsu T, Taniguchi K. Further characterization of the external urethral sphincter in spinal cord injury: study during spinal shock and evolution of responsiveness to alpha-adrenergic stimulation. J Urol 1984;131:1122–6.
48. Lemack GE, Frohman EM, Zimmern PE, et al. Urodynamic distinctions between idiopathic detrusor overactivity and detrusor overactivity secondary to multiple sclerosis. Urology 2006;67:960–4.
49. Lemack GE, Frohman E, Ramnarayan P. Women with voiding dysfunction secondary to bladder outlet dyssynergia in the setting of multiple sclerosis do not demonstrate significantly elevated intravesical pressures. Urology 2007;69:893–7.
50. Ciancio SJ, Mutchnik SE, Rivera VM, et al. Urodynamic pattern changes in multiple sclerosis. Urology 2001;57:239–45.
51. Blaivas JG, Barbalias GA. Detrusor-external sphincter dyssynergia in men with multiple sclerosis: an ominous urologic condition. J Urol 1984;131:91–4.
52. Tauber SC, Nau R, Gerber J. Systemic infections in multiple sclerosis and experimental autoimmune encephalomyelitis. Arch Physiol Biochem 2007;113:124–30.
53. Hufschmidt A, Shabarin V, Rauer S, et al. Neurological symptoms accompanying urinary tract infections. Eur Neurol 2010;63(3):180–3.
54. Metz LM, McGuinness SD, Harris C. Urinary tract infections may trigger relapse in multiple sclerosis. Axone 1998;19:67–70.
55. Rapp NS, Gilroy J, Lerner AM. Role of bacterial infection in exacerbation of multiple sclerosis. Am J Phys Med Rehabil 1995;74:415–8.
56. Urinary dysfunction and multiple sclerosis: evidence based management strategies for urinary dysfunction and multiple sclerosis. Multiple Sclerosis Council practice guidelines. Washington, DC: Paralyzed Veterans of America; 1999.
57. Porru D, Campus G, Garau A, et al. Urinary tract dysfunction in multiple sclerosis: is there a relation with disease-related parameters? Spinal Cord 1997;35:33–6.
58. Lemack GE, Hawker K, Frohman E. Incidence of upper tract abnormalities in patients with neurovesical dysfunction secondary to multiple sclerosis: analysis of risk factors at initial urologic evaluation. Urology 2005;65:854–7.
59. Krhut J, Hradílek P, Zapletalová O. Analysis of the upper urinary tract function in multiple sclerosis patients. Acta Neurol Scand 2008;118:115–9.
60. Giannantoni A, Scivoletto G, Di Stasi SM, et al. Urological dysfunctions and upper urinary tract involvement in multiple sclerosis patients. Neurourol Urodyn 1998;17:89–98.
61. Bahmanyar S, Montgomery SM, Hillert J, et al. Cancer risk among patients with multiple sclerosis and their parents. Neurology 2009;72:1170–7.
62. Rinaldi L, Perini P, Calabrese M, et al. Cyclophosphamide as second-line therapy in multiple

sclerosis: benefits and risks. Neurol Sci 2009;30 (Suppl 2):S171–3.
63. Fowler CJ, Panicker JN, Drake M, et al. A UK consensus on the management of the bladder in multiple sclerosis. J Neurol Neurosurg Psychiatry 2009;80:470–7.
64. Nygaard IE, Kreder KJ, Lepic MM, et al. Efficacy of pelvic floor muscle exercises in women with stress, urge, and mixed urinary incontinence. Am J Obstet Gynecol 1996;174(1 Pt 1):120–5.
65. De Ridder D, Ost D, Van der Aa F, et al. Conservative bladder management in advanced multiple sclerosis. Mult Scler 2005;11:694–9.
66. De Ridder D, Vermeulen C, Ketelaer P, et al. Pelvic floor rehabilitation in multiple sclerosis. Acta Neurol Belg 1999;99:61–4.
67. McClurg D, Ashe RG, Marshall K, et al. Comparison of pelvic floor muscle training, electromyography biofeedback, and neuromuscular electrical stimulation for bladder dysfunction in people with multiple sclerosis: a randomized pilot study. Neurourol Urodyn 2006;25:337–48.
68. McClurg D, Ashe RG, Lowe-Strong AS. Neuromuscular electrical stimulation and the treatment of lower urinary tract dysfunction in multiple sclerosis—a double blind, placebo controlled, randomised clinical trial. Neurourol Urodyn 2008;27: 231–7.
69. Kalsi V, Fowler CJ. Therapy insight: bladder dysfunction associated with multiple sclerosis. Nat Clin Pract Urol 2005;2:492–501.
70. Fader M, Glickman S, Haggar V, et al. Intravesical atropine compared to oral oxybutynin for neurogenic detrusor overactivity: a double-blind, randomized crossover trial. J Urol 2007;177:208–13.
71. Bennett N, O'Leary M, Patel AS, et al. Can higher doses of oxybutynin improve efficacy in neurogenic bladder? J Urol 2004;171:749–51.
72. Nicholas RS, Friede T, Hollis S, et al. Anticholinergics for urinary symptoms in multiple sclerosis. Cochrane Database Syst Rev 2009;1:CD004193.
73. Freeman RM, Adekanmi O, Waterfield MR, et al. The effect of cannabis on urge incontinence in patients with multiple sclerosis: a multicentre, randomised placebo-controlled trial (CAMS-LUTS). Int Urogynecol J Pelvic Floor Dysfunct 2006;17: 636–41.
74. O'Riordan JI, Doherty C, Javed M, et al. Do alpha-blockers have a role in lower urinary tract dysfunction in multiple sclerosis? J Urol 1995;153:1114–6.
75. Elu S, Borisov VV, Demina TL. [Tamsulosin in the treatment of detrusor-sphincter dyssynergia of the urinary bladder in patients with multiple sclerosis]. Urologia 2004;4:48–51 [in Russian].
76. Kilicarslan H, Ayan S, Vuruskan H, et al. Treatment of detrusor sphincter dyssynergia with baclofen and doxazosin. Int Urol Nephrol 2006;38:537–41.
77. Valiquette G, Herbert J, Maede-D'Alisera P, et al. Desmopressin in the management of nocturia in patients with multiple sclerosis. A double-blind, crossover trial. Arch Neurol 1996;53:1270–5.
78. Zahariou A, Karamouti M, Karagiannis G, et al. Maximal bladder capacity is a positive predictor of response to desmopressin treatment in patients with MS and nocturia. Int Urol Nephrol 2008;40: 65–9.
79. Bosma R, Wynia K, Havlíková E, et al. Efficacy of desmopressin in patients with multiple sclerosis suffering from bladder dysfunction: a meta-analysis. Acta Neurol Scand 2005;112:1–5.
80. Vahter L, Zopp I, Kreegipuu M, et al. Clean intermittent self-catheterization in persons with multiple sclerosis: the influence of cognitive dysfunction. Mult Scler 2009;15:379–84.
81. Fakas M, Souli M, Koratzanis G, et al. Effects of antimicrobial prophylaxis on asymptomatic bacteriuria and predictors of failure in patients with multiple sclerosis. J Chemother 2010;22:36–43.
82. Stoffel JT, McGuire EJ. Outcome of urethral closure in patients with neurologic impairment and complete urethral destruction. Neurourol Urodyn 2006;25:19–22.
83. Meeks JJ, Erickson BA, Helfand BT, et al. Reconstruction of urethral erosion in men with a neurogenic bladder. BJU Int 2009;103(3):378–81.
84. Wiart L, Joseph PA, Petit H, et al. The effects of capsaicin on the neurogenic hyperreflexic detrusor. A double blind placebo controlled study in patients with spinal cord disease. Preliminary results. Spinal Cord 1998;36:95–9.
85. de Sèze M, Wiart L, Joseph PA, et al. Capsaicin and neurogenic detrusor hyperreflexia: a double-blind placebo-controlled study in 20 patients with spinal cord lesions. Neurourol Urodyn 1998;17:513–23.
86. Silva C, Silva J, Ribeiro MJ, et al. Urodynamic effect of intravesical resiniferatoxin in patients with neurogenic detrusor overactivity of spinal origin: results of a double-blind randomized placebo-controlled trial. Eur Urol 2005;48:650–5.
87. de Sèze M, Wiart L, de Sèze MP, et al. Intravesical capsaicin versus resiniferatoxin for the treatment of detrusor hyperreflexia in spinal cord injured patients: a double-blind, randomized, controlled study. J Urol 2004;171(1):251–5.
88. MacDonald R, Monga M, Fink HA, et al. Neurotoxin treatments for urinary incontinence in subjects with spinal cord injury or multiple sclerosis: a systematic review of effectiveness and adverse effects. J Spinal Cord Med 2008;31:157–65.
89. Wefer B, Ehlken B, Bremer J, et al. Treatment outcomes and resource use of patients with neurogenic detrusor overactivity receiving botulinum toxin A (BOTOX(R)) therapy in Germany. World J Urol 2010;28:385–90.

90. Ehren I, Volz D, Farrelly E, et al. Efficacy and impact of botulinum toxin A on quality of life in patients with neurogenic detrusor overactivity: a randomised, placebo-controlled, double-blind study. Scand J Urol Nephrol 2007;41:335–40.
91. Gamé X, Mouracade P, Chartier-Kastler E, et al. Botulinum toxin-A (Botox) intradetrusor injections in children with neurogenic detrusor overactivity/neurogenic overactive bladder: a systematic literature review. J Pediatr Urol 2009;5(3):156–64.
92. Kalsi V, Gonzales G, Popat R, et al. Botulinum injections for the treatment of bladder symptoms of multiple sclerosis. Ann Neurol 2007;62:452–7.
93. Schurch B, Denys P, Kozma CM, et al. Botulinum toxin A improves the quality of life of patients with neurogenic urinary incontinence. Eur Urol 2007;52:850–8.
94. Schulte-Baukloh H, Schobert J, Stolze T, et al. Efficacy of botulinum-A toxin bladder injections for the treatment of neurogenic detrusor overactivity in multiple sclerosis patients: an objective and subjective analysis. Neurourol Urodyn 2006;25:110–5.
95. Popat R, Apostolidis A, Kalsi V, et al. A comparison between the response of patients with idiopathic detrusor overactivity and neurogenic detrusor overactivity to the first intradetrusor injection of botulinum-A toxin. J Urol 2005;174:984–9.
96. Gallien P, Reymann JM, Amarenco G, et al. Placebo controlled, randomised, double blind study of the effects of botulinum A toxin on detrusor sphincter dyssynergia in multiple sclerosis patients. J Neurol Neurosurg Psychiatry 2005;76:1670–6.
97. Smith CP, Nishiguchi J, O'Leary M, et al. Single-institution experience in 110 patients with botulinum toxin A injection into bladder or urethra. Urology 2005;65:37–41.
98. Lekka E, Lee LK. Successful treatment with intradetrusor botulinum-A toxin for urethral urinary leakage (catheter bypassing) in patients with end-staged multiple sclerosis and indwelling suprapubic catheters. Eur Urol 2006;50:806–9 [discussion: 809–10].
99. Schulte-Baukloh H, Bigalke H, Miller K, et al. Botulinum neurotoxin type A in urology: antibodies as a cause of therapy failure. Int J Urol 2008;15(5):407–15.
100. Marinkovic SP, Gillen LM. Sacral neuromodulation for multiple sclerosis patients with urinary retention and clean intermittent catheterization. Int Urogynecol J Pelvic Floor Dysfunct 2010;21:223–8.
101. Wallace PA, Lane FL, Noblett KL. Sacral nerve neuromodulation in patients with underlying neurologic disease. Am J Obstet Gynecol 2007;197(1):96, e1–5.
102. Chartier-Kastler EJ, Ruud Bosch JL, Perrigot M, et al. Long-term results of sacral nerve stimulation (S3) for the treatment of neurogenic refractory urge incontinence related to detrusor hyperreflexia. J Urol 2000;164:1476–80.
103. Fjorback MV, Rijkhoff N, Petersen T, et al. Event driven electrical stimulation of the dorsal penile/clitoral nerve for management of neurogenic detrusor overactivity in multiple sclerosis. Neurourol Urodyn 2006;25(4):349–55.
104. Kabay S, Kabay SC, Yucel M, et al. The clinical and urodynamic results of a 3-month percutaneous posterior tibial nerve stimulation treatment in patients with multiple sclerosis-related neurogenic bladder dysfunction. Neurourol Urodyn 2009;28:964–8.
105. Fjorback MV, van Rey FS, van der Pal F, et al. Acute urodynamic effects of posterior tibial nerve stimulation on neurogenic detrusor overactivity in patients with MS. Eur Urol 2007;51:464–70 [discussion: 471–2].
106. Fjorback MV, Van Rey FS, Rijkhoff NJ, et al. Electrical stimulation of sacral dermatomes in multiple sclerosis patients with neurogenic detrusor overactivity. Neurourol Urodyn 2007;26:525–30.
107. Gamé X, Chartier-Kastler E, Ayoub N, et al. Outcome after treatment of detrusor-sphincter dyssynergia by temporary stent. Spinal Cord 2008;46:74–7.
108. Stöhrer M, Kramer G, Goepel M, et al. Bladder autoaugmentation in adult patients with neurogenic voiding dysfunction. Spinal Cord 1997;35(7):456–62.
109. Zachoval R, Pitha J, Medova E, et al. Augmentation cystoplasty in patients with multiple sclerosis. Urol Int 2003;70:21–6.
110. Tan HJ, Stoffel J, Daignault S, et al. Ileovesicostomy for adults with neurogenic bladders: complications and potential risk factors for adverse outcomes. Neurourol Urodyn 2008;27:238–43.
111. Hellenthal NJ, Short SS, O'Connor RC, et al. Incontinent ileovesicostomy: long term outcomes and complications. Neurourol Urodyn 2009;28:483–6.
112. Gudziak MR, Tiguert R, Puri K, et al. Management of neurogenic bladder dysfunction with incontinent ileovesicostomy. J Urol 1999;54:1008–11.
113. Vanni AJ, Cohen MS, Stoffel JT. Robotic-assisted ileovesicostomy: initial results. Urology 2009;74(4):814–8.
114. Desmond AD, Shuttleworth KE. The results of urinary diversion in multiple sclerosis. Br J Urol 1977;49:495–502.

Neuromodulation and the Neurogenic Bladder

Frank N. Burks, MD, Don T. Bui, MD,
Kenneth M. Peters, MD*

KEYWORDS

- Neuromodulation • Neurogenic bladder
- Voiding dysfunction

Spinal cord injury (SCI) is a devastating event whose sequelae of paralysis, paresthesia, and bowel and bladder dysfunction have significant lifelong consequences. There are an estimated 12,000 new cases of SCI annually in the United States alone.[1] Neurogenic voiding dysfunction is a major contributor to the morbidity and mortality of SCI. Spina bifida and myelomeningocele are equally debilitating conditions that have a similar spectrum of symptoms including voiding dysfunction. Historically, renal disease has been the major cause of death in the paraplegic due to poor bladder management.[2] More recently, as a better understanding of low-pressure storage and efficient emptying has been gained, paraplegics in developed countries now die from pneumonia, septicemia, heart disease, accidents, and suicide.[3] Normal lower urinary tract function consists of low-pressure storage and voluntary, coordinated expulsion of urine. Neurogenic voiding patterns range from bladder atony to hyper-reflexia with detrusor external sphincter dyssynergia (DESD) or synergia. Uncoordinated voiding or high storage pressures can cause upper tract deterioration, while high residual urine volumes can lead to recurrent urinary infections. The use of anticholinergics and clean intermittent catheterization (CIC) has led to significant improvements in the urologic health of these patients with proven efficacy and low complication rates.[4,5] Despite these gains, persistent issues with regards to urinary tract infections, urethral strictures, upper tract deterioration, cost, and compliance continue to plague this patient population.

Neuromodulation is the electrical or physical modulation of a nerve to influence the physiologic behavior of an organ. In 1989, Tanagho and colleagues[6] pioneered the initial investigations into electrical stimulation for neuromodulation. Since this early work, neuromodulation has become an important tool in the treatment of bladder dysfunction. This article reviews the application of various electrical neuromodulation techniques to treat neurogenic bladder as well as the recent literature on surgical interventions to alleviate the symptoms of neurogenic bladder and restore normal voiding.

THE PHYSIOLOGY OF NEUROMODULATION

The exact neural mechanisms responsible for the effects of electrical neuromodulation on the lower urinary tract are unknown. A significant amount of research has focused on the effect of sacral neuromodulation (SNM) on afferent sensory nerve fibers, with the dominant theory being that electrical stimulation of these somatic afferent fibers modulates voiding and continence reflex pathways in the central nervous system (CNS).[7] The control of sensory input to the CNS is thought to work through a gate–control mechanism.[8] The gate–control theory states that noxious stimuli perception does not entirely depend on the A-delta and C-fiber sensory nerves transmitting information to the

Department of Urology, William Beaumont Hospital, 3535 West Thirteen Mile Road, Suite 438 MOB, Royal Oak, MI 48073, USA
* Corresponding author.
E-mail address: kmpeters@beaumont.edu

Urol Clin N Am 37 (2010) 559–565
doi:10.1016/j.ucl.2010.06.007
0094-0143/10/$ – see front matter

CNS, but on the pattern of peripheral nerve activity.[9] A-delta bladder afferent nerve fibers project to the pontine nuclei to provide inhibitory and excitatory input to reflexes controlling bladder and sphincter function. Afferent C-fibers within the bladder are normally thought to be mechanoinsensitive and unresponsive and thus referred to as silent C-fibers. These normally inactive C-fibers may be sensitized by inflammation or infection, thus causing activation of involuntary micturition reflexes and detrusor overactivity.[10] Sensory input from large myelinated pudendal nerve fibers may modulate erroneous bladder input conveyed by A-delta or C-fiber afferents at the gate–control level of the spinal cord. Detrusor hyper-reflexia then may be attributed to a deficiency of the inhibitory control systems involving pudendal afferent nerves. The success of electrical neuromodulation for detrusor hyper-reflexia may result from the restoration of the balance between bladder inhibitory and excitatory control systems.[11] The stimulation of urethral afferents to facilitate the micturition reflex and stimulation of the dorsal nerve of the clitoris to inhibit bladder activity have been demonstrated in animal models for SNM.[12]

Another theory behind the effectiveness for SNM for hyper-reflexia is that electrical neuromodulation may alter cortical sensory areas of the brain. Blok and colleagues[13] used positron emission tomography (PET) to evaluate regional cerebral blood flow in patients with chronic SNM and those patients with recently activated SNM. Their findings demonstrated activation of different areas of the cerebral cortex among patients with chronic and acute SNM. This finding also implies that the brain undergoes neuroplasticity during periods of long-term SNM in the areas of detrusor hyperactivity, awareness of bladder filling, the urge to void, and the timing of micturition. Other studies have used changes in somatosensory-evoked potentials before and after SNM to illustrate the cortical effects of SNM.[14]

Neuromodulation also has been used effectively for the treatment of nonobstructive urinary retention, and while the mechanism of action is not entirely clear, experimental data shed some light in this area. One such study by Schultz-Lampel and colleagues[15] investigated the effects of direct sacral nerve stimulation on detrusor contractility in cats. Their data suggested that sacral nerve stimulation at low frequencies resulted in detrusor contractions. An associated rebound effect was noted with increasing amplitude of detrusor contractions with cessation of the sacral stimulus. The authors suggest that this rebound effect may be attributed to the sacral stimulus, enabling previously inhibited bladder efferent activity and thus allowing a bladder contraction. Neuromodulation also may remedy sphincter dyssynergia and the inability to void by the alteration of afferent signals delivered to the spinal cord that affect activity and basal tone of the pelvic floor.[16]

SACRAL NERVE STIMULATION

Sacral nerve stimulation long has been a reliable form of neuromodulation for various types of lower urinary tract dysfunction including overactive bladder and nonobstructive urinary retention. These two therapeutic indications make it an attractive option for treating patients with neurogenic bladder. Lombardi and colleagues[17] described their experience with SNM in patients with an incomplete SCI suffering from neurogenic lower urinary tract symptoms with a mean follow-up of 61 months. They divided their study population into two groups, with one group consisting of patients with urinary retention (n = 13) and the other group consisting of patients with overactive bladder symptoms (n = 11). In the urinary retention group 9 of 13 (69%) patients reported a 50% improvement in baseline voiding parameters, with a significant decrease in the number of catheterizations and a significant increase in the frequency of void and voided volume. At the conclusion of the study, 38% of patients no longer required catheterization for bladder emptying. Among the patients with overactive bladder symptoms, an 80% reduction in daytime frequency was observed, with 3 out of 7 subjects with previous urge incontinence remaining completely dry during the study period. This study illustrates the dual efficacy of SNM for the spectrum of voiding dysfunction found in SCI patients. Other trials of SNM for neurogenic bladder have been less promising. Hohenfellner and colleagues[18] described their experience with SNM among patients with neurogenic bladder dysfunction. Their patient population consisted of patients with bladder storage failure due to detrusor hyper-reflexia (n = 15), failure to empty due to detrusor areflexia (n = 11), and combined bladder hypersensitivity and detrusor areflexia (n = 1), with a mean follow-up of 89 months. In eight patients (30%), symptoms of lower urinary tract dysfunction were attenuated by 50% for 54 months (range 11–96 months). After this time period, all implants became ineffective, except in one patient. This study illustrates that while SNM may be effective for neurogenic bladder dysfunction, the results may be temporary.

RISK WITH MAGNETIC RESONANCE IMAGING AFTER IMPLANT—WHEN IS IT SAFE?

As the use of sacral nerve stimulators becomes more popular worldwide, there are important safety considerations, especially with regards to magnetic resonance imaging (MRI). MRI is an important diagnostic tool for multiple medical and neurologic disorders. MRI is currently contraindicated in patients with implantable devices.[19] The possible hazards of performing MRI with an implantable device such as a sacral neuromodulator include device movement, dislocation of the neurostimulator, excessive heat to the nerve, changes in programming, and damage to the neurostimulator components. Elkelini and Hassouna[20] retrospectively reviewed histories of six patients who underwent a total of eight MRI examinations with sacral neuromodulation. Five examinations were of the brain, while three other examinations were of the cervical and thoracic vertebrae using a magnetic resonance system operating at a static magnetic field strength of 1.5 T. No patients reported any unusual symptoms during the examination, and imaging was not affected by the pulse generator located away from the imaged anatomic area. The pulse generators were turned off before MRI examination and when interrogated after the examination, no malfunctions were found. There was no change in the perception of stimulus once the pulse generator was reactivated, and follow-up voiding diaries revealed no changes in voiding parameters. Although the author's findings are encouraging, the routine use of MRI with an implanted device such as Interstim (Medtronic, Minneapolis, Minnesota) still should be used with caution.

COMPLICATIONS OF SACRAL NEUROMODULATION

Complications from SNM have been well described and are usually minor adverse events. The rate of complication ranges from 12%[21] to 53%[22] depending on the examined series. A recent article by White and colleagues[23] followed patients receiving SNM for urinary urge/frequency, urge incontinence, and urinary retention to record the incidence of adverse events and determine if there are predictive factors predisposing patients to adverse events. At a mean follow-up of 37 months, 30% of patients had experienced adverse events. Lead migration, lack of efficacy, and trauma were the most common adverse events. Significant predictors of adverse events included a history of trauma, a change in body mass index class, enrollment in a pain clinic, the duration of follow-up, and a history of adverse events.

PUDENDAL NEUROMODULATION FOR NEUROGENIC BLADDER

The pudendal nerve is a peripheral nerve that is composed mainly of afferent sensory fibers from sacral nerve roots S1, S2, and S3. Most afferent sensory fibers are contributed by S2 (60%) and S3 (35%) according to afferent activity mapping procedures.[24] Consequently, the pudendal nerve is a major contributor to bladder afferent regulation and bladder function. Pudendal nerve entrapment often leads to significant voiding dysfunction, including urinary incontinence and detrusor hyper-reflexia.[25] Because the pudendal nerve carries such a large percentage of afferent fibers, neuromodulation of the pudendal nerve is an attractive option for refractory detrusor hyperreflexia. Opisso and colleagues[26] compared patient-controlled pudendal nerve stimulation with automatic stimulation to treat neurogenic detrusor overactivity. A total of 17 patients with neurogenic detrusor overactivity underwent three cystometric filling trials. The first cystometry was used to determine bladder capacity. The second cystometry was done with automatic electrical stimulation of the pudendal nerve when the bladder reached a threshold pressure of 10 cm H_2O above the mean detrusor pressure. The third filling cystometry was done with patients controlling the pudendal stimulation and asked to begin stimulation when they could sense the onset of an uninhibited bladder contraction. Automatic and patient-controlled pudendal nerve stimulation resulted in greater bladder capacity in all subjects and inhibited more than an average of 2 detrusor contractions per filling. The authors suggest that based on their findings patients with neurogenic detrusor overactivity may be able to use patient-controlled stimulation of the pudendal nerve to increase bladder capacity and prevent uninhibited detrusor contractions. Spinelli and colleagues[27] described their experience with pudendal nerve stimulation using a device with a quadrapolar tined lead placed at Alcock canal in 15 patients with neurogenic bladder. In this study, the average number of incontinent episodes among this group of patients decreased from seven to three episodes per day. Eight patients became continent during the screening phase of the study, and four patients had a greater than 50% improvement in the number of incontinent episodes experienced per day. Urodynamic evaluation in seven patients revealed a significant increase in detrusor capacity and a decrease in maximum detrusor pressure. The authors suggest that based on these preliminary data, pudendal nerve stimulation is an effective therapeutic alternative for neurogenic overactive bladder patients who are nonresponders to antimuscarinic drugs and in whom traditional sacral neuromodulation has had poor results. The authors also point out that the minimally invasive nature of pudendal nerve stimulation using the quadrapolar tined lead is an attractive alternative to more invasive procedures such as bladder augmentation. Currently at the authors' institution, the most common indication for pudendal neuromodulation is for patients who have had failure of sacral neuromodulation. The placement of the lead is done via a posterior approach and requires electrophysiologic monitoring of the pudendal nerve action potentials intraoperatively to confirm pudendal stimulation.

NEUROMODULATION OF THE POSTERIOR TIBIAL NERVE FOR NEUROGENIC BLADDER

The posterior tibial nerve is a peripheral mixed sensory–motor nerve that originates from spinal roots L4 through S3, which also contribute directly to sensory and motor control of the urinary bladder and pelvic floor. Stimulation of the posterior tibial nerve was pioneered by Stoller and colleagues[28] with the introduction of a nerve stimulator, which delivers electrical stimulation to the posterior tibial nerve via a 34-gauge needle just cephalad to the medial malleolus. Multiple studies have demonstrated that posterior tibial nerve stimulation (PTNS) shows some efficacy in treating symptoms of detrusor hyperactivity[29,30] and altering urodynamic findings in patients with overactive bladder.[31] A recent article prospectively examined the use of PTNS among children with voiding dysfunction with 2 years of follow-up.[32] Of the 43 patients in the trial, 12 had neurogenic bladder due to spinal dysraphism at the sacral level. Patients were evaluated before and after PTNS with a voiding diary and noninvasive voiding measurements. Relief of lower urinary tract symptoms was significantly greater in patients with non-neurogenic bladder than those with neurogenic bladder (78% vs 14%). The authors suggest that the variable results among patients with neurogenic bladder resulting from spinal dysraphism may be due to the variable neural lesions found among these patients and that improved patient selection might lead to more impressive results.

FINETECH-BRINDLEY POSTERIOR/ANTERIOR STIMULATOR

Research regarding electrical stimulation to improve micturition in SCI patients has been on going for the last 50 years. In 1969, Brindley developed a device to stimulate sacral roots at the level of the cauda equina. The first Brindley stimulator was implanted in a patient in 1978. Although the first implants did not involve posterior sacral rhizotomy, lesions to these nerves during surgery led to the advantage of leaving the patient's bladder completely areflexic and restoring normal bladder compliance and curing reflex incontinence. Subsequently, placement of the Brindley stimulator was combined with sacral posterior rhizotomy.[33] The deinnervation step is skipped in cases of genital sensation and reflex erections. Over a retrospective review of 500 patients with a Brindley stimulator, 411 were still in use with the patients pleased.[34] Ergon and colleagues[33] reviewed their experience with 93 SCI patients with sacral anterior root stimulators combined with posterior sacral rhizotomy. They reported that 83 patients used their stimulators for micturition, and 82 were fully continent. The major limitation to this form of neuromodulation is that it requires an intact neural pathway between the sacral cord nuclei of the pelvic nerve and the bladder.[35] This is not always the case, especially in children with lap belt injuries that result in lower motor neuron lesions.

HEMILAMINECTOMY AND VENTRAL ROOT MICROANASTOMOSIS, THE XIAO PROCEDURE

Kilvington first described the idea of bladder reinnervation in 1907, but he failed to demonstrate any response after lumbar-to-sacral reinnervation in a canine model. Subsequently, Xiao's landmark study with rats confirmed the assumption that the efferent root of a somatic reflex arc could regenerate into the autonomic efferent root that controls the bladder.[36] A total of 24 rats underwent a lateral hemilaminectomy. After transaction of L4 and L6 ventral roots, the proximal end of the L4 ventral root was attached to the L6 ventral root. After allowing 3 months for axonal regrowth, 15 rats underwent neurophysiological experiments, and 6 rats had horseradish peroxidase (HRP) neural tracing studies. The final three rats were saved for a year for long-term observation. Of the 15 rats, 12 were viable for study, and in all of them, a bladder detrusor contraction was elicited by L4 electrical stimulation. This contraction generated an average of 38 plus or minus 7 cm H_2O of intravesical pressure. The HRP tracings demonstrate histologically the successful regeneration of somatic motor axons into an autonomic efferent root. In four rats, somatic motor neurons in the L4 ventral horn were positively labeled with the HRP, while the remaining two had traces in left pelvic ganglia neuron axons. The long-term specimens proved the functionality of the reflex arc. Electrical stimulation of the distal sciatic nerve caused a bladder contraction, as did scratching of the L4 dermatome. This then was tested on six cats by intradural microanastomosis of the left L7 ventral root (VR) to the S1 VR. This created a skin-CNS-bladder reflex that uses the cutaneous afferent signal to trigger the micturition reflex arc.[37] After 7 months of recovery, cutaneous stimulation of the L7 dermatome created a strong detrusor contraction that resulted in an elevation of bladder pressure (45 ± 8 cm H_2O). Of note, the four long-term subjects exhibited no consequential motor deficits.

The success in animal models encouraged human trials. Xiao described how he created a somatic-CNS-autonomic pathway in 15 patients with hyper-reflexic neurogenic bladders and DESD secondary to complete suprasacral SCI.[38] A microanastomosis was made between the L5 ventral root and the S2\3 ventral root to allow the motor axons to reinnervate the autonomic preganglionic nerves. These patients were followed with postoperative urodynamic evaluations for an average of 3 years of postoperatively. In 10 of the 15 patients, bladder function, including storage and emptying, was recovered. Similar to the animal models, cutaneous stimulation of the appropriate dermatome instigated the skin-CNS-bladder reflex, causing voiding. Interestingly, 4 of these 10 patients had resolution of their hyper-reflexia with DESD to normal voiding with low postvoid residuals. The remaining six had no change in their DESD, but they were able to use the new reflex to successfully void with low residuals. The Xiao procedure then was performed on 20 children with spina bifida.[39] Preoperatively, 14 had an areflexic detrusor with small bladder capacity, open urethral outlet and incontinence. The remaining six suffered from hyper-reflexic bladder with DESD, similar to the suprasacral SCI patients. Seventeen of the 20 patients (85%) recovered acceptable bladder storage and function. Those with atonic bladders had an average increase of bladder capacity of 94 mL to 177 mL and a decrease in postvoid residuals (70 mL–24 mL), with only two patients failing to see any improvement. Of those with DESD, five were able to void spontaneously with a significant decrease in mean detrusor pressure. Five of the 20 patients developed a motor deficit in L4 or L5, ranging from slight muscle weakness to visible foot drop. No other complications were reported. It was noted that from a technical perspective, the spina bifida cases were more challenging than SCI secondary to the abnormal neuroanatomy.[39]

NORTH AMERICAN EXPERIENCE WITH THE XIAO PROCEDURE

There have been attempts to replicate the Xiao procedure in the United States. The first trial involved two traumatic SCI patients, a complete T6 and T11, respectively, causing neurogenic detrusor overactivity with DESD. Prior to the nerve rerouting surgery, the patients were being managed by CIC and anticholinergics. An intradural anastomosis was unilaterally made between the ventral root of L5 to S3. At 6 months after operating, detrusor contractions were elicited via cutaneous L5 stimulation in both patients as well as a significant decrease in detrusor overactivity. By the 15-month follow-up, both patients were completely off anticholinergics and CIC. Cystometrogram studies show that L5 stimulation generates a detrusor contraction of 59 cm H_2O, a Q max of 8 cc/s with no DESD. Voided volume was 150 cc, and postvoid residual was 200 cc/s. There were no significant complications in this small cohort.[40]

A larger study was performed in a group of nine spina bifida patients, mean age 8 years (range 6–37 years). All patients were on a CIC regimen preoperatively and underwent a rigorous neurologic, urologic, urodynamic, and lumbar–sacral examination before surgery. The Xiao anastomosis was made between the unilateral ventral lumbar root and S3. There were no surgical complications. At 1 year after operating, seven out of nine patients were able to generate at least a 10 cm H_2O rise in detrusor pressure with cutaneous stimulation of the dermatome. Mean PVR was 119 cc (range 10–380 cc), Qmax of 10 cc\s (range 4–25 cc/s). No patient achieved complete urinary continence, and only two were able to completely stop CIC. Two unintended benefits were noted. First, the bowel function of the patients improved significantly. The procedure has changed their quality of life enough to the point where seven out of nine would undergo it again. The other peculiar anecdote is a return of bladder sensation. Many subjects reported the return of early filling sensation of both the bowel and bladder. Unfortunately, one patient did suffer from foot drop that significantly worsened her gait. There were no other significant neurologic complications at 1-year follow-up, and changes in bowel and bladder function continue to improve with longer follow-up.[41]

SUMMARY

Neuromodulation is changing the management of voiding dysfunction. Techniques using both electrical and mechanical stimulation are being researched to help correct the underlying bladder and bowel dysfunction. Advances in neuromodulation techniques may allow the clinician to abandon irreversible destructive/reconstructive procedures such as bladder augmentation and urinary diversion. Further research into this field is needed to expand understanding of neurourology and improve the treatment of patients.

REFERENCES

1. Rabchaevsky AG, Smith GM. Therapeutic interventions following mammalian spinal cord injury. Arch Neurol 2001;58:721–6.
2. Hackler RH. A 25-year prospective mortality in the spinal cord injured patient: comparison with the long-term living paraplegic. J Urol 1977;117:486–92.
3. Soden RJ, Walsh J, Middleton JW, et al. Causes of death after spinal cord injury. Spinal Cord 2000;38:604–10.
4. Lapides J, Diokno A, Silber S, et al. Clean intermittent self-catheterization in the treatment of urinary tract disease. J Urol 1972;107:458–65.
5. Weld KJ, Dmochowski RR. Effect of bladder management on urological complications in spinal cord injured patients. J Urol 2000;163(3):768–72.
6. Tanagho EA, Schmidt RA, Orvis BR. Neural stimulation for control of voiding dysfunction: a preliminary report in 22 patients with serious neuropathic voiding disorders. J Urol 1989;142:340–5.
7. Leng WW, Chancellor MB. How sacral nerve stimulation neuromodulation works. Urol Clin North Am 2005;23:11–8.
8. Alo KM, Holsheimer J. New trends in neuromodulation for the management of neuropathic pain. Neurosurgery 2002;50:690–703.
9. Melzack R, Wall PD. Pain mechanisms: a new theory. Science 1965;150:971–9.
10. Cheng CL, Ma CP, de Groat WC. Effect of capsaicin on micturition and associated reflexes in rats. Am J Physiol 1993;265:132–8.
11. van der Pal F, Heesakkers J. Current opinion on the working mechanisms of neuromodulation in the treatment of lower urinary tract dysfunction. Curr Opin Urol 2006;16:261–7.
12. Vignes JR, Deloire MS, Petry KG. Animal models of sacral neuromodulation for detrusor overactivity. Neurourol Urodyn 2009;28:8–12.
13. Blok BF, Groen J, Bosch JL, et al. Different brain effects during chronic and acute sacral neuromodulation in urge incontinent patients with implanted neurostimulators. BJU Int 2006;98:1238–43.
14. Malaguti S, Spinelli M, Giardiello G, et al. Neurophysiological evidence may predict the outcome of sacral neuromodulation. J Urol 2003;170:2323–6.
15. Schult-Lampel D, Jiang C, Lindstrom S, et al. Experimental results on mechanisms of action of electrical neuromodulation in chronic urinary retention. World J Urol 1998;16:301–4.
16. Schmidt RA, Jonas U, Oleson KA, et al. Sacral nerve stimulation for treatment of refractory urinary urge incontinence. J Urol 1999;62:352–7.
17. Lombardi G, Del Popolo G. Clinical outcome of sacral neuromodulation in incomplete spinal cord injured patients suffering from neurogenic lower urinary tract symptoms. Spinal Cord 2009;47:486–91.
18. Hohenfellner M, Humke J, Hampel C, et al. Chronic sacral neuromodulation for treatment of neurogenic baldder dysfunction: long term results with unilateral implants. Urology 2001;58(6):887–92.
19. Shellock FG, Kanal E. SMRI reoprt: policies, guidelines and recommendations for MR imaging safety and patient management. J Magn Reson Imaging 1992;2:247–8.
20. Elkelinin MS, Hassouna MM. Safety of MRI at 1.5 Tesla in patients with implanted sacral nerve neurostimulator. Eur Urol 2006;50:311–6.
21. Gaynor-Krupnick DM, Dwyer NT, Rittenmeyer H, et al. Evaluation and management of malfunctioning sacral neuromodulatior. Urology 2006;67:246–9.
22. Sutherland SE, Lavers A, Carlson A, et al. Sacral nerve stimulation for voiding dysfunction: one institution's 11-year experience. Neurourol Urodyn 2007;26:19–28.
23. White WM, Mobley JD, Doggweiler R, et al. Incidence and predictors of complications with sacral neuromodulation. Urology 2009;73:731–5.
24. Huang JC, Deletis V, Vodusek DB, et al. Preservation of pudendal affferents in sacral rhizotomies. Neurosurgery 1997;41:411–5.
25. Beco J, Climov D, Bex M. Pudendal nerve decompression in perineology: a case series. BMC Surg 2004;4:15.
26. Opisso E, Borau A, Rodrigues A, et al. Patient controlled versus automatic stimulation of pudendal nerve affferents to treat neurogenic detrusor overactivity. J Urol 2008;180:1404–8.
27. Spinelli M, Malaguti S, Giardiello G, et al. A new minimally invasive procedure for pudendal nerve stimulation to treat neurogenic bladder: description of the method and preliminary data. Neurourol Urodyn 2005;24:305–9.
28. Cooperberg MR, Stoller ML. Percutaneous neuromodulation. Urol Clin North Am 2005;32:71–8.
29. Govier F, Litwiller S, Nitti V, et al. Percutaneous afferent modulation for the refractory over active bladder: results of a multicenter study. J Urol 2001;165:1193–8.
30. vanBalken MR, Vandoninck V, Gisolf K, et al. Posterior tibial nerve stimulation as neuromodulatory treatment of lower urinary tract dysfunction. J Urol 2001;166:914–8.
31. Klingler HC, Pycha A, Schmidbauer J, et al. Use of peripheral neuromodulation of the S3 region for treatment of detrusor overactivity: a urodynamic-based study. Urology 2000;56:766–71.
32. Capitanucci ML, Camanni D, Demelas F, et al. Long-term efficacy of percutaneous tibial nerve

stimulation for different types of lower urinary tract dysfunction in children. J Urol 2009;184(4): 2056–61.
33. Egon G, Barat M, Colombel P, et al. Implantation of anterior sacral root stimulators combined with posterior sacral rhizotomy in spinal injury patients. World J Urol 1998;16:342–9.
34. Brindley GS. The first 500 patients with sacral anterior root stimulator implants: general description. Paraplegia 1994;32:795–805.
35. Fischer J, Madersbacher H, Zechberger J, et al. Sacral anterior root stimulation to promote micturition in transverse spinal cord lesions. Zentralbl Neurochir 1993;54:77–9.
36. Xiao CG, Godec CJ. A possible new reflex pathway for micturation after spinal cord injury. Paraplegia 1994;32:300–7.
37. Xiao CG, De Groat W, Godec CJ. Skin-CNS-bladder reflex pathway for micturition after spinal cord injury and its underlying mechanisms. J Urol 1999;162: 936–42.
38. Xiao CG, Du M, Dai C, et al. An artificial somatic–central nervous system–autonomic reflex pathway for controllable micturition after spinal cord injury: preliminary results in 15 patients. J Urol 2003;170:1237–41.
39. Xiao CG, Du M, Li B, et al. An artificial somatic-autonomic reflex pathway procedure for bladder control in children with spina bifida. J Urol 2005; 173:2112–6.
40. Kelly C, Xiao CG, Weiner H, et al. Creation of a somatic–autonomic reflex pathway for treatment of neurogenic bladder in patients with spinal cord injury: preliminary results of first 2 USA patients [abstract]. J Urol 2005;173:1132A.
41. Peters K, Xiao CG, Girdler B, et al. One-year outcomes with lumbar to sacral nerve rerouting in spina bifida [abstract]. J Urol 2009;181(4):310–1.

Botulinum Toxin Therapy for Neurogenic Detrusor Overactivity

Marc C. Smaldone, MD, Benjamin T. Ristau, MD, Wendy W. Leng, MD*

KEYWORDS

- Botulinum toxin • Bladder dysfunction • Neurogenic
- Detrusor overactivity • Overactive bladder

The overactive bladder (OAB) condition is a symptom complex characterized by urinary urgency with or without urge urinary incontinence (UUI), and is often associated with frequency and nocturia. Overall, OAB prevalence in the United States and European adult population is estimated to be 11.8%.[1] OAB is not specific to any one condition. However, based on clinical convention; OAB may then be further classified as neurogenic or idiopathic. When OAB occurs in association with a known underlying neurologic pathology such as spinal cord injury (SCI) or multiple sclerosis (MS), it is classified as neurogenic OAB. When there is no evidence of any identifiable neurologic disorder, it is classified as idiopathic OAB.

OAB is a clinical diagnosis. By contrast, detrusor overactivity (DO) describes the common urodynamic testing observation in this population, whereby involuntary detrusor contractions become evident during the bladder-filling phase.[2] For the purposes of this discussion of neurogenic bladder dysfunction, the authors use the term neurogenic detrusor overactivity (NDO).

Research demonstrates the significant impairment to quality of life (QOL)[3] by OAB as well as its added burden of increasing health care costs.[4] While the OAB condition clearly affects QOL for all sufferers, the subset of patients with NDO can be even more disadvantaged by virtue of their neurologic deficits.

Moreover, neurogenic bladder dysfunction has the distinct potential to cause long-term renal failure. The neural and/or myogenic deficits may gradually compromise the bladder's storage function, otherwise known as bladder compliance. Such insidious, asymptomatic deterioration of the neurogenic bladder's compliance reflects a gradual loss of the lower urinary tract's ability to store increasing volume at the same low ambient pressure. With the ensuing increase in intravesical storage pressure, the lower urinary tract often responds by provoking random urethral leakage as a means to vent a high-pressure chamber.[5] However, in some instances where the system fails to satisfactorily vent the high-pressure chamber, the sustained high pressures transmit upstream to the renal pelvis. Over time, this sustained high-pressure transmission to the renal pelvis causes deterioration of glomerular filtration and eventual renal failure. This well-characterized pathophysiologic process poses a dangerously asymptomatic phenomenon for the NDO population.[6]

Typically, first-line therapy for idiopathic OAB is conservative in nature, encompassing behavioral techniques, pelvic physiotherapy, and antimuscarinic pharmacotherapy. While conservative

Department of Urology, University of Pittsburgh School of Medicine, Suite 700, Kaufmann Building, 3471 5th Avenue, Pittsburgh, PA 15213, USA
* Corresponding author.
E-mail address: lengww@upmc.edu

Urol Clin N Am 37 (2010) 567–580
doi:10.1016/j.ucl.2010.06.001
0094-0143/10/$ – see front matter

therapies are likewise reasonable for first-line management of NDO, the chances of successful incontinence control are greatly hindered by patient disabilities and the underlying neurologic defects within the complex micturition circuit. In other words, a significant fraction of NDO patients derive insufficient bladder control with conservative treatment strategies. Moreover, this patient population disproportionately suffers more overall QOL impairment with their lower urinary tract dysfunction.[7]

A growing body of evidence suggests that intravesical injection of botulinum neurotoxin (BTX) is an efficacious, minimally invasive alternative to more traditional surgical therapies (such as bladder augmentation or urinary diversion) in patients with NDO who are intolerant or refractory to pharmacotherapy. Alternative intravesical agents currently being evaluated include antimuscarinic agents (oxybutynin, atropine), local anesthetics (lidocaine, bupivacaine), and vanilloids (capsaicin, resiniferatoxin), but randomized, placebo-controlled evidence demonstrating safety and efficacy is currently lacking.[8] The objective of this review is to provide a focused summary of the current body of literature investigating the safety and efficacy of bladder BTX injection in patients with NDO.

MECHANISM OF ACTION

Botulinum toxin, produced by the gram-positive anaerobic bacterium *Clostridium botulinum* and first isolated by van Ermengem in 1897,[9] is among the most potent biologic neurotoxins known to man. Structurally composed of a 150-kDa amino acid di-chain molecule consisting of a light (50 kDa) and heavy (100 kDa) chain linked by a disulfide bond, BTX's primary mechanism of action is inhibition of acetylcholine release at the presynaptic cholinergic junction.[10] BTX's high selectivity for cholinergic synapses results in targeted blockade of cholinergic transmission, which when targeted to striated muscle induces muscle paresis.[11] More specifically, BTX reduces type Ia/II intrafusal muscle fiber afferent conduction, affecting the spinal stretch reflex and decreasing muscle tone and contractility without affecting muscle strength.[12,13] Investigators have postulated recently that, in addition a direct effect on detrusor motor innervation, BTX may also affect afferent nervous transmission via the inhibition of acetylcholine, adenosine triphosphate (ATP), glutamate, nerve growth factor, and substance P, and a reduction in the axonal expression of nerve capsaicin and purinergic (P2X) receptors.[14] Thus, it seems likely that BTX also modulates intrinsic bladder reflexes, resulting in central desensitization and a decrease in urgency (**Fig. 1**).[15] Duration of effect is likely multifactorial as well; mechanisms including chemical denervation followed by axonal regeneration[16] as well as functional motor suppression through neurotransmitter inhibitory effects[14] have been proposed.

SEROTYPES, TOXICITIES, AND COMMERCIAL PREPARATIONS

Seven BTX serotypes have been isolated, 2 of which (BTX-A and BTX-B) have been investigated in treating bladder dysfunction. The most commonly investigated serotype worldwide, BTX-A received Food and Drug Administration (FDA) approval for therapeutic treatment of strabismus and blepharospasm in 1989, cervical dystonia in 2000, and cosmetic treatment of glabellar wrinkles in 2002. In a recent review of all adverse events (AE) reported to the FDA since BTX-A was licensed in 1989, Cote and colleagues[17] described 217 serious AE, including 28 deaths. All occurred during therapeutic administration but the investigators concluded that it was impossible to determine a causal relationship between the reported mortalities and BTX administration. Additional AE included dysphagia (12%), muscle weakness (6%), allergic reaction (5%), and flu-like syndrome (5%). During cosmetic use, the investigators reported primarily nonserious AE and no deaths, most commonly lack of effect (63%), injection site reaction (19%), and ptosis (11%). Although the FDA has not yet approved BTX for urologic use in the United States, BTX is currently being investigated for urologic indications in clinical trials worldwide. At present, BTX is available as 3 major commercial preparations: Botox (BTX-A; Allergan, Irvine, CA, USA), Dysport (BTX-A; Ipsen, Slough, UK), and Myobloc (BTX-B; Solstice Neurosciences, San Diego, CA, USA).[18] Each of these preparations has different dosages, safety profiles, and efficacy profiles, and cannot be used interchangeably. In the only head to head comparison to date, Grosse and colleagues[18] performed an open-label, observational case-control study comparing a single treatment session of Dysport (500 U, 750 U, 1000 U) and Botox (300 U), finding no differences in therapeutic parameters between groups.

RATIONALE FOR TREATMENT

Since the 1980s, clinicians have been using BTX to treat neurologic disorders, such as blepharospasm, strabismus, focal dystonias, muscle spasms and spasticity, axillary hyperhidrosis,

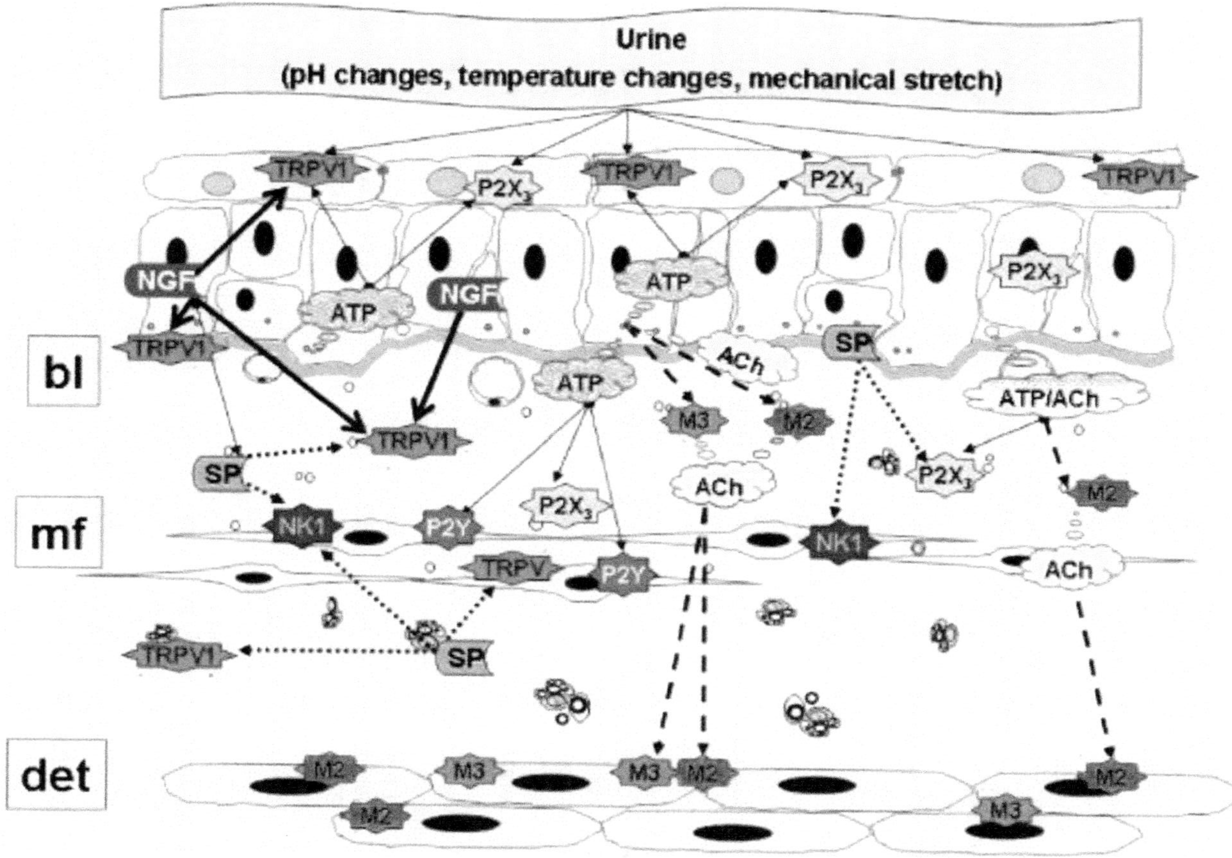

Fig. 1. The structural components of the human bladder wall including the basal lamina (bl), myofibroblast layer (mf), and detrusor muscle (det). Superimposed are the known or proposed location of receptors and sites of neuropeptide/growth factor release involved in bladder mechanosensation. All connections identified by arrows are thought to be upregulated in detrusor overactivity and may be reduced with the peripheral afferent desensitization that follows injection of botulinum toxin. Thin solid arrows, a proposed pathway where urothelial vesicular ATP release activates P2X2-P2Y receptors or potentiates the response of TRPV1 receptors to irritative stimuli; thin dashed arrows, proposed pathways where vesicular acetylcholine (ACh) release from urothelial nerve terminals activates detrusor muscle muscarinic ACh receptors; thick dashed arrows, proposed pathways where substance P (SP) acts on NK1 receptors on the myofibroblast layer or potentiates the activation of TRPV1-P2X3 receptors in sub-urothelial afferents; thick solid arrows, nerve growth factor (NGF) is thought to affect the expression of TRPV1. (*Reprinted from* Apostolidis A, Dasgupta P, Fowler CJ. Proposed mechanism for the efficacy of injected botulinum toxin in the treatment of human detrusor overactivity. Eur Urol 2006;49[4]:647; Copyright [2006], with permission from Elsevier.)

and achalasia.[19] The initial application of BTX-A to the lower urinary tract targeted patients with detrusor external sphincter dyssynergia (DESD). BTX-A was injected into the urethral sphincter with the intention of weakening the urethral striated musculature enough to reduce urethral pressures, and in turn, to decrease bladder voiding pressures and post-void residual volumes (PVR).[20,21] However, over the past decade the off-label use of BTX in treating detrusor overactivity (both neurogenic and idiopathic) has become a source of significant interest among urologists. Demonstrating posttreatment reduction in detrusor pressures during voiding and involuntary contractions has provided evidence of BTX's effect on detrusor motor innervation,[22,23] and patient-reported reduction in sensation of urgency lends support to a dual afferent mechanism of action as well.[24]

With current investigations expanding the utility of BTX even further to include interstitial cystitis, pelvic floor dysfunction, and prostatic applications; there is currently a wide variation in reported dosages, injection techniques, and follow-up protocols being used. This pattern has led to current efforts to create evidence-based guidelines governing BTX use.[25] However, it is clear that the dosage, number, and site of injection should be tailored to the individual needs of each patient based on etiology of bladder dysfunction. In patients with idiopathic DO or interstitial cystitis, the goals of treatment are to provide symptomatic relief, while avoiding negative side effects such as straining to void and urinary retention. However, in addition to improving QOL, the primary goals of BTX bladder injection in patients with neurogenic DO are to improve urodynamic storage parameters and minimize the risk of renal impairment.[26] For these reasons, it is imperative that all NDO patients being evaluated for BTX injection undergo pretreatment urodynamics assessment. Because BTX chemical denervation is reversible over time, the main disadvantage of BTX injection is the need to undergo repeat injections. Fortunately, there is now evidence to suggest that repeat treatment is equally efficacious even after several injections.[27]

DOSAGE, CONCENTRATION, AND INJECTION TECHNIQUE

Published investigations to date have utilized varying doses, volumes, and injection target sites. These variations make systematic comparative assessment of the safety and efficacy of BTX difficult. A recent systematic literature review of BTX injection protocol characteristics reported that typically 300 U BTX-A (range 100–400 U) was injected in 30 sites (range 15–40) of 10 U/mL (range 6.7–25 U/mL) in the detrusor, with most investigators preferring to spare the trigone. Injection is typically performed under cystoscopic guidance (flexible or rigid), and can be performed under several types of anesthesia (none, local, spinal, or general).[28]

Injection doses ranging from 100 to 400 U (Botox), and 500 to 1000 SU (Dysport) have been reported in published studies to date. The 300-U dose is the most consistently used across series, although isolated series have reported 100, 200, and 400 U. Although few studies have specifically investigated variable dosing, similar improvement has been reported regardless of total dose with respect to both subjective and objective outcomes.[29] However, determining which dose offers maximum clinical effect with the least risk has not yet been determined. When an initial evaluation of BTX-A injection using 200 U and 300 U in 31 patients with NDO revealed that 2 patients receiving 200 U failed to show clinical improvement, Schurch and colleagues[23] concluded that 300 U was the optimal treatment dose.[30] However, prospective comparison of 200 U and 300 U in 59 patients with NDO showed significant subjective and objective improvement in all patients, with no differences between the 2 study arms. A recent meta-analysis of 8 randomized controlled OAB trials including BTX in at least one treatment arm reported that while low doses of BTX (100–150 U) appeared to have beneficial effects, higher doses (300 U) may be more effective. The investigators concluded that the optimal dose of BTX for efficacy and safety can not be determined until more definitive clinical trial data are available.[31] A majority of investigations to date have utilized injection volumes ranging from 0.1 to 0.5 mL (6.7–25 U/mL)/injection site.[28] Based on animal models, it has been proposed that larger dilution volumes will result in greater suburothelial diffusion with an increased treatment effect.[32] However, this has not been demonstrated clinically, and there are concerns that larger volumes increase the potential for serosal extravasation and increased patient discomfort.[29]

Although various techniques have been described, BTX injection is commonly performed under intravenous sedation or local anesthesia following administration of prophylactic antibiotics. In the operating room setting with the patient in the lithotomy position, a 21F rigid cystoscope and collagen injection needle are used to create a submucosal bleb under direct vision. If a flexible cystoscope is used, a longer needle and/or sheath for stabilization may be necessary.[33] With increasing experience, the injection technique has been uneventfully performed in the office setting, using a flexible cystoscope under local anesthesia. This approach may facilitate cost reduction and avoidance of anesthetic risks.[29]

With endoscopic guidance, toxin is injected via 15 to 40 evenly distributed intramural injection sites including the bladder base and posterolateral walls (**Fig. 2**). As a general principle, the bladder dome is excluded because of concerns regarding intraperitoneal perforation and bowel injury, and the trigone is spared to avoid inducing vesicoureteral reflux.[26] In cases of DO arising from non-neurogenic cause and/or in patients with isolated pain/sensory components, recent protocols have included trigonal injection, with good results.[33]

TREATMENT OUTCOMES

A recent systematic literature review identified 18 studies investigating the use of BTX in patients with NDO. In this aggregate population of 698 patients, 83% had NDO with urinary incontinence refractory to high doses of anticholinergic therapy. Based on the aggregate outcomes, the investigators concluded that BTX detrusor injections provide a clinically significant benefit in adults with NDO and incontinence/OAB refractory to antimuscarinics.[28] However, of the studies included in the systematic review, only 3 retrospective studies examined clinical series larger than 75 patients (all retrospective),[34–36] and only 3 other studies were prospectively randomized with a control arm.[23,37,38] The majority consisted of small open-labeled studies of less than 50 patients (**Table 1**).[18,22,26,27,30,39–52]

In a large multi-institutional retrospective series, Reitz and colleagues[35] reported significant increases in mean cystometric bladder capacity ($P<.0001$), mean reflex volume ($P<.01$), and decreased mean voiding pressures ($P<.0001$) in 231 patients with NDO. Patients were treated with 300 U BTX-A in 30 trigone-sparing injection sites; and with 36 week follow-up, patients reported considerably reduced anticholinergic drug dose requirements and high subjective satisfaction rates, with no injection related complications or side effects. Stoehrer and colleagues[36] reported the results of BTX-A detrusor injections in 216 patients with NDO, comparing maximal detrusor pressure, detrusor compliance, reflex volume, cystometric capacity, as well as use of anticholinergic agents and patient satisfaction at 6 weeks and 6 months after treatment. Using either 300 U of Botox or 750 U of Dysport, the investigators reported a significant improvement in all urodynamic parameters as well as incontinence rates and decreased anticholinergic use, but no significant differences were noted when comparing the 2 BTX-A preparations. Recently, Del Popolo and colleagues[34] reported their findings using 1000 U, 750 U, and 500 U of BTX-A (Dysport) in 199 patients with spinal cord lesions and refractory NDO. Following urodynamic evaluation at baseline, then 3, 6, and 12 months post injection; significant improvements were noted in maximum

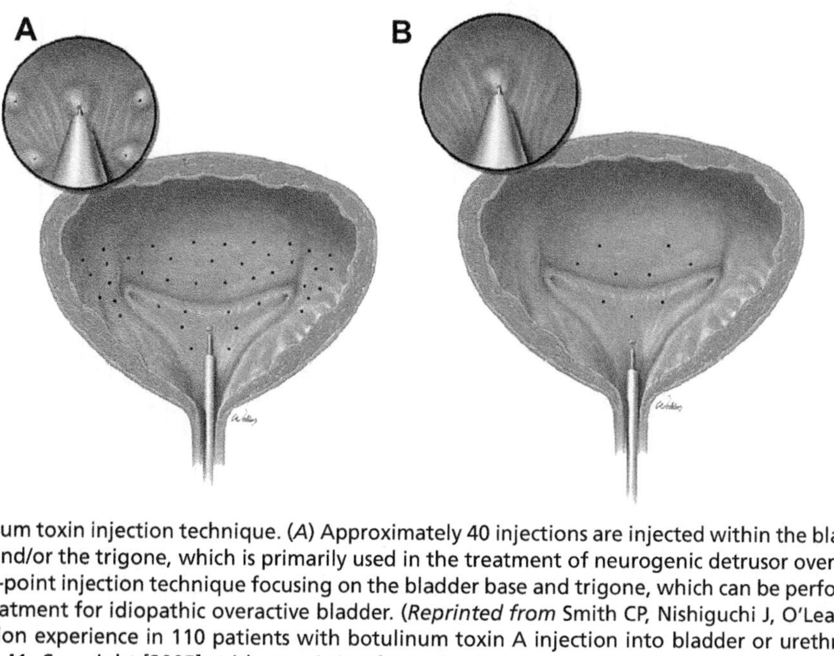

Fig. 2. Botulinum toxin injection technique. (*A*) Approximately 40 injections are injected within the bladder base, lateral walls, and/or the trigone, which is primarily used in the treatment of neurogenic detrusor overactivity. (*B*) A modified 10-point injection technique focusing on the bladder base and trigone, which can be performed as an outpatient treatment for idiopathic overactive bladder. (*Reprinted from* Smith CP, Nishiguchi J, O'Leary M, et al. Single-institution experience in 110 patients with botulinum toxin A injection into bladder or urethra. Urology 2005;65[1]:37–41; Copyright [2005], with permission from Elsevier.)

Table 1
Clinical and urodynamic findings in large retrospective or prospective series of BTX-A injection for neurogenic detrusor overactivity

Authors	Study Design (N)	BTX-A Preparation Dose (U)	No. of Injections	Incontinence Episodes/24 h	$Pdet_{max}$ (cm H_2O)	MCC (ml)	Compliance (mL/cm H_2O)	Mean Follow-Up (wk)	Adverse Events (%)
Mean change from baseline (%)									
Retrospective Studies									
Reitz et al[35]	MI (231)	Botox 300	30	73% continent 27% some improvement	−31 (51)[d]	148 (35)[d]	40 (125)[d] at 6 wk 19 (59) at 36 wk	36	N/A
Del Popolo et al[34]	SI (199)	Dysport 500 (23%), 750 (53%), 1000 (24%)	20	Decreased IEs at 4 wk[d] Decreased pads/condoms at 4 wk[d]	N/A	182 (80)[c]	N/A	48	Hyposthenia (2.5)
Stoehrer et al[36]	SI (216)	Botox 300 Dysport 750	Botox 30 Dysport 25	>80% continent with CIC	−31.1 (56)[d]	98 (33)[d]	17 (73) at 6 wk[d] 8.6 (37) at 24 wk	24	Weakness (1) Dysphagia (0.5) Dysarthria (0.5)
Prospective Studies									
Schurch et al[23]	RPC (59)	Botox 200, 300	30				N/A	24	UTI (26.3)
	Placebo (21)			−0.1 (3)	1.4 (16)	41.6 (16)			Injection site pain (5) UTI (14)
	BTX 200 U (19)			−1.1 (58)[a]	−38.7(67)[a,e]	174.2[a] (67)			UTI (32)
	BTX 300 U (19)			−0.9[a,e] (32)	−35.5[a,e] (32)	92.9[a,e] (32)			Injection site pain (11) UTI (21)
Giannantoni et al[38]	RACC (75)	Botox 300	30				N/A	112	
	RTX (35)			−2.8 (57)[c]	−8.6 (10)	93.4 (40)[b]			
	BTX (40)			−4.0[c,e] (77)	−32.9 (44)[b]	134.6 (54)[b,e]			
Ehren et al[37]	RPC (31)	Dysport 500	25				N/A	26	
	Placebo (14)			N/A	−12 (21)	10 (4)			0
	BTX (17)				−52 (77)[c,e]	180 (62)[c,e]			Hematuria (6)

Abbreviations: BTX, botulinum toxin; CIC, clean intermittent catheterization; IE, incontinence episodes; MCC, maximum cystometric capacity; MI, multi-institutional; N/A, not available; $Pdet_{max}$, maximum detrusor pressure; RACC, randomized, active comparator-controlled; RPC, randomized, placebo-controlled; RTX, resiniferatoxin; SI, single institution; UTI, urinary tract infection.

[a] *P*<.05.
[b] *P*<.01.
[c] *P*<.001.
[d] *P*<.0001.
[e] Significant versus placebo or treatment arm.

bladder capacity, reflex volume, bladder compliance, and pad usage ($P<.001$). Of note, there were no significant differences in therapeutic effect or duration of effect when comparing the differing dosing regimens.

In a double-blinded, randomized, placebo-controlled, 3-arm study comparing 200 U BTX-A, 300 U BTX-A, and placebo in 59 patients with NDO (90% SCI, 10% MS) requiring clean intermittent catheterization (CIC), Schurch and colleagues[23] investigated frequency of urinary incontinence, maximum cystometric capacity (MCC), reflex detrusor volume, and maximum detrusor pressure via patient voiding diary and urodynamic assessment at 24 weeks post injection. The investigators reported significant improvement in QOL (Incontinence Quality of Life questionnaire), posttreatment decreases in incontinence episodes (IE), and improvement in urodynamic bladder function in both BTX treatment groups ($P<.05$) from the first evaluation at week 2 to the end of the 24-week study when compared with baseline. The reported side effects with BTX use were minimal and symptom improvement was similar in the 200 U and 300 U dosing regimen groups, with no significant improvement noted in the placebo arm. Giannantoni and colleagues[38] randomized 75 patients with SCI and refractory NDO to a 2-arm controlled trial comparing intravesical instillation of resiniferatoxin (RTX) dissolved in normal saline (N = 40) and 30 trigone-sparing bladder injections of 300 U BTX-A diluted in 30 mL normal saline (N = 35). Clinical assessment and urodynamics were performed at baseline, then 6, 12, and 24 months post treatment. The investigators reported significant reductions in mean catheterization rate and IE, as well as significant increases in mean first involuntary detrusor contraction and mean maximum bladder capacity at all time points in both treatment groups. Although side effects were not reported with either treatment, the investigators did note a significant benefit with BTX compared with RTX regarding number of IE per 24 hours and maximum detrusor pressure. In the most recent prospective study to date, Ehren and colleagues[37] randomized 31 patients with NDO to a single treatment of 500 U BTX-A (Dysport) versus placebo using urodynamic parameters (6, 12, and 26 weeks), QOL, IE, and intake of rescue tolterodine as outcome measures. A significantly lower intake of tolterodine ($P = .003$), increased cystometric capacity at 6 ($P<.001$) and 12 ($P = .026$) weeks, decreased maximum detrusor pressure ($P<.01$), and decreased IE ($P<.01$) were found in the BTX treatment arm. The consensus from these reports suggests that BTX achieves measurable urodynamic and subjective improvement in NDO patients with minimal negative sequelae. However, repeat injections are necessary to achieve a sustained response. Although contemporary series differ with regard to study methodology and injection protocols, here the authors summarize and quantify the reported outcomes within the broad categories of subjective patient-reported outcome measures and objective urodynamic parameters.

CLINICAL PARAMETERS: PATIENT-REPORTED

Incontinence Episodes

In a review of 18 studies, Karsenty and colleagues[28] reported that the mean pre-BTX treatment IE per 24 hours ranged from 1.9 to 5.4 (it must be noted that a large proportion of these patients were concurrently managed with CIC). Up to 26 weeks following injection, the percentage reduction in the mean number of IE from baseline ranged from 60% to 80%,[22,23,38,40,45,46] and reported total continence rates ranged from 42% to 87%,[39,50] although the rate of full return to continence was only 8% in patients with NDO due to cerebrovascular accident.[50] Of the randomized controlled evidence available, Schurch and colleagues[23] reported significant incontinence improvement in both treatment arms compared with baseline (1.9–0.8 IE/24 h BTX 200 U, $P<.05$; 2.8–1.9 IE/24 h BTX 300 U, $P<.05$), as well as with the placebo arm at 24 weeks after treatment (3.0–2.9 IE/24 h). Likewise, at 26 weeks post treatment, Giannantoni and colleagues[38] reported significant improvement in both treatment arms compared with baseline (4.9–2.1 IE/24 h RTX, $P<.001$; 5.2–1.2 IE/24 h BTX, $P<.001$) with a more dramatic effect observed in the BTX treatment arm. Confirming these observations, Ehren and colleagues[37] reported significant differences in the number of days with leakage following detrusor injection with BTX-A or placebo, at less than 6 weeks ($P<.001$), 7 to 12 weeks ($P = .002$), and 13 to 26 weeks ($P = .01$).

Antimuscarinic Use

Several case series also document the impact of BTX therapy on antimuscarinic use.[22,30,35,36,39,40] Of the prospective cohorts, Ehren and colleagues[37] reported the dose of "rescue drug" tolterodine as a primary outcome measure, and found that patients undergoing a single treatment of BTX-A used significantly less tolterodine over a 26-week period compared with the placebo arm ($P = .003$). In a retrospective cohort of 216 patients, Stoehrer and colleagues[36] reported that 50% of patients discontinued anticholinergic medications after 6 weeks, and at 6 months 35% still had not resumed therapy. In their retrospective series of 231 patients with NDO, Reitz and colleagues[35] reported that of the 163 patients on anticholinergic medications prior to BTX therapy, concomitant anticholinergic medication could be discontinued in 45 patients (25.6%) and was considerably reduced in 118 patients (72.4%) following treatment. Summarizing the available literature, Karsenty and colleagues[28] reported that antimuscarinic agents could be discontinued in 28% to 58% of patients following BTX therapy,[22,30,35] and the requirement could be substantially reduced in the remaining patients.

Quality of Life

QOL outcomes are more difficult to interpret, as a wide variety of QOL instruments, including the Urogenital Distress Inventory (UDI-6),[45,52] Symptom Severity Index (SSI),[52] Qualiveen questionnaire,[37] Symptom Impact Index (SII),[52] Incontinence QOL questionnaire (I-QOL),[23] Visual Analog Scale (VAS),[34] and International Prostate Symptom Score (I-PSS),[49] have been utilized in series investigating use of BTX in patients with NDO. Using the I-QOL questionnaire, Schurch and colleagues[23] prospectively assessed QOL following BTX injection, and observed robust improvements compared with baseline at all time points up to 24 weeks. There were no significant QOL differences between 200 U and 300 U BTX-A dosing regimens, but both groups had significantly higher QOL scores when compared with placebo at all time points. Utilizing the Qualiveen questionnaire, Ehren and colleagues[37] noted that patients treated with BTX-A reported a significantly higher QOL related to bother with incontinence that lasted throughout the study period (26 weeks). In their systematic review, Karsenty and colleagues[28] reported a percent mean change in QOL ranging from 35% to 61% following BTX therapy when data from all QOL instruments were aggregated. Hori and colleagues[44] recently assessed posttreatment satisfaction with a 5 minute telephone interview in 72 patients with SCI and NDO who had received at least one BTX injection. Patients reported a mean satisfaction score of 6.2 on a scale from 1 to 10 (1, not satisfied; 10, very satisfied), and 90% of patients replied that they would consider continuing with BTX injection therapy as a long-term treatment option.

URODYNAMIC OUTCOME MEASURES

Maximum Detrusor Pressure

Despite heterogeneous methodology and injection protocols, the majority of BTX studies demonstrate significant improvements from baseline in urodynamic parameters, namely maximum detrusor pressure ($Pdet_{max}$), MCC, and reflex detrusor volume (RDV) in patients with NDO. Reflecting recent European consensus, Apostolidis and colleagues reported that across 25 studies, the mean decrease in $Pdet_{max}$ was 44%,[25] ranging from 5% to 83%.[1,18,22,23,26,30,31,34–43,45–53] Prospectively evaluating 59 patients with 24 weeks of follow-up, Schurch and colleagues[23] reported a significant change from mean baseline $Pdet_{max}$ in both the BTX 200 U (77.0–48.8 cm H_2O, $P<.05$) and BTX 300 U (92.6–55.2 cm H_2O, $P<.05$) treatment arms. Moreover, the mean percent change from baseline in both arms (−50% BTX 200 U, −38% BTX 300 U) were significant improvements compared with the placebo group (+2%). Compared with baseline values in 75 patients, Giannantoni reported a significant decrease in mean $Pdet_{max}$ in the BTX arm (74.9–42.0 cm H_2O, $P<.01$), which was proved significant when compared with those patients in the RTX treatment arm (mean percent change from baseline, −10 RTX vs −44 BTX, $P<.01$).[38] Prospectively evaluating 31 patients, Ehren and colleagues[37] reported that the BTX-A treatment group had significantly lower $Pdet_{max}$ values at 6 ($P<.001$), 12 ($P = .02$), and 26 weeks ($P = .003$). When examining the total body of available literature including the results from open-labeled studies, following BTX treatment mean maximal $Pdet_{max}$ was reduced to less than 40 cm H_2O (range 20–59 cm H_2O) in a majority of studies,[28] which has reached consensus as the threshold value for protection of the upper urinary tract.[54] It must be taken into account that traditionally $Pdet_{max}$ refers to voiding pressures, and many patients in the NDO population do not void. Thus $Pdet_{max}$ as an individual parameter must be interpreted with caution, and should be utilized in conjunction with other urodynamic parameters such as bladder compliance.

Maximum Cystometric Capacity

The observed reduction in $Pdet_{max}$ was accompanied by an increase in MCC in most reports. Schurch and colleagues[23] reported a significant increase from baseline in both the BTX 200 U arm (260.2–440.9 mL, $P<.05$) and BTX 300 U arms (293.6–398.2 mL, $P<.05$) respectively, both of which were significant improvements compared with placebo (mean percent change vs baseline 67 BTX 200 U, 32 BTX 300 U, 16 placebo, $P<.05$). Giannantoni and colleagues[38] reported a similar improvement in both the RTX (235.6–329.0 mL, $P<.01$) and BTX (249.8–384.4 mL,

$P<.01$) arms of their prospective investigation, although the mean percent change compared with baseline was more dramatic in the BTX treatment group (40 RTX vs 54 BTX, $P<.005$). Ehren observed a similar effect with MCC significantly increasing at both 6 ($P<.001$) and 12 ($P = .03$) weeks. Yet this difference was no longer statistically significant at 26 weeks.[37] Systematically evaluating results from 25 studies, a mean increase in MCC of 85% has been reported,[25] ranging from 11% to 303% across published series.[22,23,26,30,34–38,40–43,45–50,52]

Bladder Compliance

As previously described, the neurogenic bladder population is particularly vulnerable to gradual deterioration of bladder storage capability. This insidious decrease of bladder compliance can result in long-term renal failure. Thus, serial bladder compliance assessment serves as an important surveillance tool to protect upper tract function. Because low bladder compliance can identify a particularly high-risk neurogenic bladder population who are often refractory to traditional therapies, some early studies investigating BTX bladder injection specifically excluded this subset. However, with early investigations demonstrating promising efficacy; subsequent studies have specifically examined the impact of BTX in patients with NDO and low bladder compliance.

In their systematic literature review, Karsenty and colleagues[28] reported that mean bladder compliance increased with BTX treatment. Yet not surprisingly, the observed duration of improved bladder compliance correlated with the overall self-limited effectiveness of BTX injection.[30,35,46–48] Of the larger retrospective studies, Reitz and colleagues[35] reported a mean increase in bladder compliance at 12 weeks (32–72 mL/cm H_2O, $P<.0001$), which declined by the 36-week time point (32–51 mL/cm H_2O, $P>.05$). Stoehrer and colleagues[36] reported a similar initial mean increase in compliance at 6 weeks (23.1–40 mL/cm H_2O, $P<.00001$), but this response was also not durable beyond 24 weeks (mean change at 24 weeks, 23.1–31.7 mL/cm, $P>.05$). In a small cohort specifically investigating BTX efficacy in 10 NDO patients with abnormally low bladder compliance (baseline 6.5 mL/cm H_2O), Klaphajone and colleagues[48] reported a consistent increase in compliance at 6 (mean change 6.7 mL/cm H_2O, $P<.05$) and 16 weeks (7.3 mL/cm H_2O, $P<.05$), although the effect had diminished by 36 weeks. From these results, the investigators concluded that BTX injections are effective even in patients with very low compliance, but that repeat injections may be necessary after 16 weeks to maintain a durable effect on low bladder compliance.

TREATMENT EFFECT AND EFFICACY OF REPEAT THERAPY

The exact onset of BTX treatment response remains unclear. In most studies, voiding diary collection and urodynamic parameters were not measured until 4 to 6 weeks following injection. For this reason, most series reporting treatment onset have based their results on subjective patient response. Via telephone interview or clinic visit, Smith and colleagues[26] reported that time to maximal efficacy was observed between 7 and 30 days following injection. In a more formal investigation, Rapp and colleagues[55] sent self-report questionnaires to 35 patients undergoing BTX injection for OAB, evaluating time to first response and time to maximum symptomatic improvement. Patients reported a mean time to symptom improvement of 5.3 days (range 1–14) post injection with maximum symptom improvement at a mean of 8.3 days (range 2–20). Symptom improvement has not been specifically characterized in the NDO patient population, as sensory deficits would certainly affect subjective reporting. However, Schurch and colleagues[23] reported significant improvement in both subjective and objective urodynamic parameters in NDO patients within 2 weeks following injection, reaching a maximum effect between 2 and 6 weeks.

Studies evaluating treatment duration have primarily used the number of IE per 24 hours to determine the need for repeat therapy. Karsenty and colleagues[46] retrospectively reviewed a series of 17 NDO patients who had received at least 3 BTX (mean 5.4) injections. The mean time interval between BTX injections ranged between 7.6 and 9.1 months. This observed treatment duration has been substantiated by some retrospective reports,[38] whereas others describe shorter periods of efficacy of merely 2 to 3 months, particularly in patients with decreased bladder compliance.[35,48] Several studies have investigated the long-term efficacy of repeat BTX injection for NDO.[27,41,46,56] In their evaluation of 66 patients with NDO, Grosse and colleagues[56] found similar improvement in urodynamic parameters after each repeat injection with Botox 300 U or Dysport 750 U, reporting that the interval between repeat injections did not significantly change with time (average of 9–11 months, $P = .6$). Reitz and colleagues[27] followed 20 consecutive NDO patients receiving at least 5 BTX injections, and on serial urodynamic assessment observed that clinical improvements in MCC, $Pdet_{max}$, and compliance did not change over time. In the most comprehensive series to date, Giannantoni and colleagues[41] followed 17 patients with SCI and NDO managed with BTX injection therapy for 6 years, with clinical evaluation, urodynamics, imaging of the upper tract, and QOL assessment performed annually. At final analysis, they reported a significant increase in MCC ($P<.001$) and a significant decrease in $Pdet_{max}$ ($P<.01$), with 88.2% of patients reporting complete continence. From these data, it is possible to conclude that repeat BTX detrusor injection is efficacious for NDO. However, due to the small retrospective nature of these studies, it remains unclear what proportion of patients will develop BTX resistance and associated treatment failure. In fact, development of BTX-A antibodies has been demonstrated and has been implicated in cases of BTX therapy failure.[57] Concern for BTX-A resistance has resulted in the investigation of BTX-B in the treatment of urologic disorders. Initial evaluations in de novo patients[58] and BTX-A failures[59,60] demonstrate encouraging subjective and urodynamic improvement but with a shorter duration of effect (6 weeks to 6 months). Thus, at this time, use of BTX-B remains unproven.

SAFETY

Reported significant side effects with BTX bladder injection are exceedingly uncommon, and in general BTX injection is very well tolerated. Although there is no uniform documentation system, the most commonly reported AE include injection site pain, procedure-related urinary tract infection (UTI) (2%–32%), mild hematuria (2%–21%), and an increase in PVR, which at times results in urinary retention (0%–33%) or de novo CIC (6%–88%).[28] With extended follow-up, hydronephrosis and vesicoureteral reflux have been detected in rare instances, but have been self-limited in nature.[41] Due to the paralytic mechanism of botulinum neurotoxin, theoretical concerns for systemic effects exist. However, to date there have been no reports of severe systemic reactions such as respiratory paralysis. Hyposthenia has been reported in scattered series,[34] but these events have been transient, lasting from 2 weeks to 2 months. Although there is no evidence of dose-related side effects with BTX bladder therapy, some investigators have reported initial clinical experiences with dose modification as low as 100 U in an attempt to reduce the risks of therapy.[61] However, as of yet there is no current consensus as to which candidates would benefit from lower dose therapy.

BTX INJECTION FOR NDO IN CHILDREN

The most common underlying pathology for NDO in the pediatric population is myelomeningocele (93%), followed by spinal cord tumors and trauma.[62] First-line therapies for NDO in the pediatric population include antimuscarinic pharmacotherapy and CIC, but 10% to 15% of patients will prove to have refractory disease or severe systemic side effects.[63] During the last 10 years, intravesical BTX has emerged as an alternative treatment option to bladder augmentation or incontinent urinary diversion for children with NDO refractory to traditional therapies.

A recent systematic review identified 6 small open-label studies[64–69] encompassing 108 children (mean age 9.8 years) with NDO managed with CIC who were treated with BTX injection from 2002 to 2006.[70] Injection protocols consisted of 30 to 50 injections of 5 to 12 U/kg BTX with a maximum total dose of 300 to 360 U, and the majority of procedures were performed under general anesthesia. Follow-up was variable, but was typically reported at 4- to 12-week intervals up to 26 weeks. Two studies evaluated the efficacy of reinjection, at 6 to 9 months[64] and at 1 year,[66] respectively.

The primary outcome measure of continence was quantified by the mean incontinence score.[71] BTX injection resulted in a mean 40% to 80% reduction from baseline,[65–67,69] and 65% to 87% of children became completely continent between catheterizations.[70] Improvement of urodynamic parameters was demonstrated with BTX injection as well. All 6 studies showed a significant reduction in $Pdet_{max}$[64–69] (percentage mean reduction from baseline 33%–55%).[64,68–70] The observed reduction in $Pdet_{max}$ closely corresponded with an increase in MCC (percentage increase from baseline ranging from 35% to 80%), RDV (percentage increase from baseline ranging from 84% to 314%), and bladder compliance (percentage increase from baseline ranging from 58% to 180%).[70] Similar to adult BTX series, clinical efficacy was noted within 2 weeks from injection, and these benefits were noted to persist for 3 to 6 months.[66,68] The efficacy of repeat injection therapy has also been demonstrated in children, with the mean time interval between injection treatments ranging from 6.3 to 9.6 months.[64,67] BTX injections were well tolerated in all series, with no evidence of systemic AE or muscle weakness. The most common AE reported was procedure-related UTI in 7% to 20% of patients.[70] Similar to adult NDO populations, detrusor BTX injection has been shown to have beneficial clinical and urodynamic effects in children refractory to conservative therapies.

ADDITIONAL APPLICATIONS

Detrusor External Sphincter Dyssynergia

DESD, defined as an involuntary contraction of the striated external sphincter during detrusor contraction, is classically observed in patients with central nervous system lesions between the sacral spinal cord and the brain stem (SCI, MS, and so forth). Traditional treatment modalities have included CIC, external sphincterotomy, balloon dilation of the external sphincter, and prosthetic urethral stent placement.[72] Urethral sphincter BTX injection has been proposed as a minimally invasive, reversible therapeutic option for DESD with the goal of decreasing sustained high voiding pressures to reduce the risk of damage to the upper tracts.[26]

First reported in 1988,[20] urethral sphincter BTX therapeutic results are largely derived from small open-labeled studies. These series are difficult to compare because of differing injection protocols using varying formulations and dilutions. A recent systematic review reported that urethral BTX injection resulted in a 21% to 48% reduction from baseline maximal urethral pressure, and 7% to 41% reduction of maximal detrusor voiding pressure. Yet despite treatment, the maximal detrusor voiding pressure following injection therapy remained 40 mm H_2O or more in several of these studies.[73] In a small double-blinded, placebo-controlled crossover study, Dykstra and Sidi[74] investigated urethral BTX-A injection in 5 patients (140–240 U), reporting a 34% reduction in maximal detrusor voiding pressure, 31% reduction in maximal urethral pressure, and a 40% reduction in PVR. Despite demonstrating a benefit, the study's small sample makes it difficult to draw definitive conclusions. In a multicenter, randomized, double-blinded, placebo-controlled trial, Gallien and colleagues[75] compared the efficacy of urethral injection of 100 U BTX-A to placebo saline injection in 96 patients with DESD. The investigators reported a significant reduction in maximal detrusor pressure compared with placebo (21%, $P = .02$), but no significant differences between groups with respect to maximal urethral pressure or PVR. While urethral BTX injection remains an intriguing minimally invasive therapeutic option, further prospective studies evaluating its long-term effects on voiding pressures are necessary before widespread utilization in patients with DESD.

Future Directions

Due to the successful utilization of botulinum toxin in the lower urinary tract, investigators have started to explore the promise of BTX injection for an expanded spectrum of urologic conditions. BTX injection has been investigated as a therapeutic option for patients with detrusor hypocontractility or idiopathic voiding dysfunction, as a means of reducing urethral resistance in order to decrease the need to catheterize.[76] Postulating that botulinum toxin may reverse the sphincter-induced detrusor-inhibition reflex in addition to paralyzing sphincter motor end plates,[73] BTX injection has been proposed as a potential treatment option for such voiding dysfunctions as urethral overactivity and pelvic floor spasticity.[26] Laboratory evidence suggesting an effect on afferent sensory innervation[77] shows great potential in the treatment of refractory urgency,[78] lower urinary tract symptoms in association with benign prostatic hypertrophy,[79] prostatitis/urethritis,[80] and interstitial cystitis.[26] BTX injection has also been used in the treatment of pubovaginal sling retention[81] as well as urethral stricture disease that has failed visual urethrotomy.[82] Although these applications are promising and show intriguing preliminary data, these studies represent off-label utilizations that are still only investigational at this time. Further large-scale trials are needed to validate these preliminary findings, before the lower urinary tract applications of BTX can be expanded.

SUMMARY

Bladder botulinum toxin injection appears to have beneficial qualitative and quantitative effects in patients with NDO refractory to antimuscarinic therapy. Injection therapy is well tolerated with minimal risk of systemic AE. However, questions remain regarding ultimate durability of efficacy despite encouraging results with repeat injection therapy. The current body of evidence is limited by study methodology as well as significant variations in injection technique, BTX dosages, and concentrations utilized. Ongoing global randomized, controlled trials will help to establish standardized injection protocols, confirm efficacy and safety, and discern the optimal dose to achieve a durable response in this complex patient population.

REFERENCES

1. Irwin DE, Milsom I, Hunskaar S, et al. Population-based survey of urinary incontinence, overactive bladder, and other lower urinary tract symptoms in five countries: results of the EPIC study. Eur Urol 2006;50(6):1306–14 [discussion: 1314–5].
2. Abrams P, Cardozo L, Fall M, et al. The standardisation of terminology in lower urinary tract function:

report from the standardisation sub-committee of the International Continence Society. Urology 2003;61 (1):37–49.
3. Coyne KS, Sexton CC, Irwin DE, et al. The impact of overactive bladder, incontinence and other lower urinary tract symptoms on quality of life, work productivity, sexuality and emotional well-being in men and women: results from the EPIC study. BJU Int 2008;101(11):1388–95.
4. Kannan H, Radican L, Turpin RS, et al. Burden of illness associated with lower urinary tract symptoms including overactive bladder/urinary incontinence. Urology 2009;74(1):34–8.
5. Wan J, McGuire EJ, Bloom DA, et al. Stress leak point pressure: a diagnostic tool for incontinent children. J Urol 1993;150(2 Pt 2):700–2.
6. McGuire EJ, Woodside JR, Borden TA, et al. Prognostic value of urodynamic testing in myelodysplastic patients. J Urol 1981;126(2):205–9.
7. Wyndaele JJ, Kovindha A, Madersbacher H, et al. Neurologic urinary incontinence. Neurourol Urodyn 2010;29(1):159–64.
8. Reitz A, Schurch B. Intravesical therapy options for neurogenic detrusor overactivity. Spinal Cord 2004; 42(5):267–72.
9. van Ermengem E. Ueber einen neuen anaeroben bacillus und seine beziehungen zum botulismus. Zeitsch Hyg Infekt 1897;26:1–56 [in German].
10. Simpson LL. The origin, structure, and pharmacological activity of botulinum toxin. Pharmacol Rev 1981;33(3):155–88.
11. Dressler D, Saberi FA, Barbosa ER. Botulinum toxin: mechanisms of action. Arq Neuropsiquiatr 2005;63 (1):180–5.
12. Duchen LW. Changes in motor innervation and cholinesterase localization induced by botulinum toxin in skeletal muscle of the mouse: differences between fast and slow muscles. J Neurol Neurosurg Psychiatr 1970;33(1):40–54.
13. Schiavo G, Rossetto O, Catsicas S, et al. Identification of the nerve terminal targets of botulinum neurotoxin serotypes A, D, and E. J Biol Chem 1993;268 (32):23784–7.
14. Apostolidis A, Dasgupta P, Fowler CJ. Proposed mechanism for the efficacy of injected botulinum toxin in the treatment of human detrusor overactivity. Eur Urol 2006;49(4):644–50.
15. Smith CP, Radziszewski P, Borkowski A, et al. Botulinum toxin a has antinociceptive effects in treating interstitial cystitis. Urology 2004;64(5):871–5 [discussion: 875].
16. Haferkamp A, Schurch B, Reitz A, et al. Lack of ultrastructural detrusor changes following endoscopic injection of botulinum toxin type a in overactive neurogenic bladder. Eur Urol 2004;46(6):784–91.
17. Cote TR, Mohan AK, Polder JA, et al. Botulinum toxin type A injections: adverse events reported to the US Food and Drug Administration in therapeutic and cosmetic cases. J Am Acad Dermatol 2005;53(3): 407–15.
18. Grosse J, Kramer G, Jakse G. Comparing two types of botulinum-A toxin detrusor injections in patients with severe neurogenic detrusor overactivity: a case-control study. BJU Int 2009;104(5):651–6.
19. Truong DD, Stenner A, Reichel G. Current clinical applications of botulinum toxin. Curr Pharm Des 2009;15(31):3671–80.
20. Dykstra DD, Sidi AA, Scott AB, et al. Effects of botulinum A toxin on detrusor-sphincter dyssynergia in spinal cord injury patients. J Urol 1988;139(5): 919–22.
21. Schurch B, Hauri D, Rodic B, et al. Botulinum-A toxin as a treatment of detrusor-sphincter dyssynergia: a prospective study in 24 spinal cord injury patients. J Urol 1996;155(3):1023–9.
22. Popat R, Apostolidis A, Kalsi V, et al. A comparison between the response of patients with idiopathic detrusor overactivity and neurogenic detrusor overactivity to the first intradetrusor injection of botulinum-A toxin. J Urol 2005;174(3):984–9.
23. Schurch B, de Seze M, Denys P, et al. Botulinum toxin type a is a safe and effective treatment for neurogenic urinary incontinence: results of a single treatment, randomized, placebo controlled 6-month study. J Urol 2005;174(1):196–200.
24. Schmid DM, Sauermann P, Werner M, et al. Experience with 100 cases treated with botulinum-A toxin injections in the detrusor muscle for idiopathic overactive bladder syndrome refractory to anticholinergics. J Urol 2006;176(1):177–85.
25. Apostolidis A, Dasgupta P, Denys P, et al. Recommendations on the use of botulinum toxin in the treatment of lower urinary tract disorders and pelvic floor dysfunctions: a European consensus report. Eur Urol 2009;55(1):100–19.
26. Smith CP, Nishiguchi J, O'Leary M, et al. Single-institution experience in 110 patients with botulinum toxin A injection into bladder or urethra. Urology 2005;65(1):37–41.
27. Reitz A, Denys P, Fermanian C, et al. Do repeat intradetrusor botulinum toxin type a injections yield valuable results? Clinical and urodynamic results after five injections in patients with neurogenic detrusor overactivity. Eur Urol 2007;52(6):1729–35.
28. Karsenty G, Denys P, Amarenco G, et al. Botulinum toxin A (Botox) intradetrusor injections in adults with neurogenic detrusor overactivity/neurogenic overactive bladder: a systematic literature review. Eur Urol 2008;53(2):275–87.
29. Rapp DE, Lucioni A, Bales GT. Botulinum toxin injection: a review of injection principles and protocols. Int Braz J Urol 2007;33(2):132–41.
30. Schurch B, Stohrer M, Kramer G, et al. Botulinum-A toxin for treating detrusor hyperreflexia in spinal

cord injured patients: a new alternative to anticholinergic drugs? Preliminary results. J Urol 2000;164(3 Pt 1):692–7.
31. Duthie J, Wilson DI, Herbison GP, et al. Botulinum toxin injections for adults with overactive bladder syndrome. Cochrane Database Syst Rev 2007;(3): CD005493.
32. Kim HS, Hwang JH, Jeong ST, et al. Effect of muscle activity and botulinum toxin dilution volume on muscle paralysis. Dev Med Child Neurol 2003;45 (3):200–6.
33. Smith CP, Chancellor MB. Simplified bladder botulinum-toxin delivery technique using flexible cystoscope and 10 sites of injection. J Endourol 2005;19(7):880–2.
34. Del Popolo G, Filocamo MT, Li Marzi V, et al. Neurogenic detrusor overactivity treated with English botulinum toxin a: 8-year experience of one single centre. Eur Urol 2008;53(5):1013–9.
35. Reitz A, Stohrer M, Kramer G, et al. European experience of 200 cases treated with botulinum-A toxin injections into the detrusor muscle for urinary incontinence due to neurogenic detrusor overactivity. Eur Urol 2004;45(4):510–5.
36. Stoehrer M, Wolff A, Kramer G, et al. Treatment of neurogenic detrusor overactivity with botulinum toxin A: the first seven years. Urol Int 2009;83(4): 379–85.
37. Ehren I, Volz D, Farrelly E, et al. Efficacy and impact of botulinum toxin A on quality of life in patients with neurogenic detrusor overactivity: a randomised, placebo-controlled, double-blind study. Scand J Urol Nephrol 2007;41(4):335–40.
38. Giannantoni A, Mearini E, Di Stasi SM, et al. New therapeutic options for refractory neurogenic detrusor overactivity. Minerva Urol Nefrol 2004;56(1): 79–87.
39. Bagi P, Biering-Sorensen F. Botulinum toxin A for treatment of neurogenic detrusor overactivity and incontinence in patients with spinal cord lesions. Scand J Urol Nephrol 2004;38(6):495–8.
40. Giannantoni A, Di Stasi SM, Nardicchi V, et al. Botulinum-A toxin injections into the detrusor muscle decrease nerve growth factor bladder tissue levels in patients with neurogenic detrusor overactivity. J Urol 2006;175(6):2341–4.
41. Giannantoni A, Mearini E, Del Zingaro M, et al. Six-year follow-up of botulinum toxin A intradetrusorial injections in patients with refractory neurogenic detrusor overactivity: clinical and urodynamic results. Eur Urol 2009;55(3):705–11.
42. Hajebrahimi S, Altaweel W, Cadoret J, et al. Efficacy of botulinum-A toxin in adults with neurogenic overactive bladder: initial results. Can J Urol 2005;12 (1):2543–6.
43. Harper M, Popat RB, Dasgupta R, et al. A minimally invasive technique for outpatient local anaesthetic administration of intradetrusor botulinum toxin in intractable detrusor overactivity. BJU Int 2003;92 (3):325–6.
44. Hori S, Patki P, Attar KH, et al. Patients' perspective of botulinum toxin-A as a long-term treatment option for neurogenic detrusor overactivity secondary to spinal cord injury. BJU Int 2009;104(2):216–20.
45. Kalsi V, Apostolidis A, Popat R, et al. Quality of life changes in patients with neurogenic versus idiopathic detrusor overactivity after intradetrusor injections of botulinum neurotoxin type A and correlations with lower urinary tract symptoms and urodynamic changes. Eur Urol 2006;49(3):528–35.
46. Karsenty G, Reitz A, Lindemann G, et al. Persistence of therapeutic effect after repeated injections of botulinum toxin type A to treat incontinence due to neurogenic detrusor overactivity. Urology 2006;68 (6):1193–7.
47. Kessler TM, Danuser H, Schumacher M, et al. Botulinum A toxin injections into the detrusor: an effective treatment in idiopathic and neurogenic detrusor overactivity? Neurourol Urodyn 2005;24(3):231–6.
48. Klaphajone J, Kitisomprayoonkul W, Sriplakit S. Botulinum toxin type A injections for treating neurogenic detrusor overactivity combined with low-compliance bladder in patients with spinal cord lesions. Arch Phys Med Rehabil 2005;86(11): 2114–8.
49. Kuo HC. Urodynamic evidence of effectiveness of botulinum A toxin injection in treatment of detrusor overactivity refractory to anticholinergic agents. Urology 2004;63(5):868–72.
50. Kuo HC. Therapeutic effects of suburothelial injection of botulinum a toxin for neurogenic detrusor overactivity due to chronic cerebrovascular accident and spinal cord lesions. Urology 2006;67(2):232–6.
51. Pannek J, Gocking K, Bersch U. Long-term effects of repeated intradetrusor botulinum neurotoxin A injections on detrusor function in patients with neurogenic bladder dysfunction. BJU Int 2009;104(9): 1246–50.
52. Schulte-Baukloh H, Schobert J, Stolze T, et al. Efficacy of botulinum-A toxin bladder injections for the treatment of neurogenic detrusor overactivity in multiple sclerosis patients: an objective and subjective analysis. Neurourol Urodyn 2006;25(2):110–5.
53. Kalsi V, Popat RB, Apostolidis A, et al. Cost-consequence analysis evaluating the use of botulinum neurotoxin-A in patients with detrusor overactivity based on clinical outcomes observed at a single UK centre. Eur Urol 2006;49(3):519–27.
54. McGuire EJ, Savastano JA. Urodynamics and management of the neuropathic bladder in spinal cord injury patients. J Am Paraplegia Soc 1985;8 (2):28–32.
55. Rapp DE, Lucioni A, Katz EE, et al. Use of botulinum-A toxin for the treatment of refractory

overactive bladder symptoms: an initial experience. Urology 2004;63(6):1071–5.
56. Grosse J, Kramer G, Stohrer M. Success of repeat detrusor injections of botulinum a toxin in patients with severe neurogenic detrusor overactivity and incontinence. Eur Urol 2005;47(5):653–9.
57. Schulte-Baukloh H, Bigalke H, Miller K, et al. Botulinum neurotoxin type A in urology: antibodies as a cause of therapy failure. Int J Urol 2008;15(5): 407–15 [discussion: 415].
58. Dykstra D, Enriquez A, Valley M. Treatment of overactive bladder with botulinum toxin type B: a pilot study. Int Urogynecol J Pelvic Floor Dysfunct 2003; 14(6):424–6.
59. Pistolesi D, Selli C, Rossi B, et al. Botulinum toxin type B for type A resistant bladder spasticity. J Urol 2004;171(2 Pt 1):802–3.
60. Reitz A, Schurch B. Botulinum toxin type B injection for management of type A resistant neurogenic detrusor overactivity. J Urol 2004;171(2 Pt 1):804 [discussion: 804–5].
61. Cohen BL, Barboglio P, Rodriguez D, et al. Preliminary results of a dose-finding study for botulinum toxin-A in patients with idiopathic overactive bladder: 100 versus 150 units. Neurourol Urodyn 2009;28(3):205–8.
62. Carr MC. Bladder management for patients with myelodysplasia. Surg Clin North Am 2006;86(2): 515–23, xi-xii.
63. Hernandez RD, Hurwitz RS, Foote JE, et al. Nonsurgical management of threatened upper urinary tracts and incontinence in children with myelomeningocele. J Urol 1994;152(5 Pt 1):1582–5.
64. Altaweel W, Jednack R, Bilodeau C, et al. Repeated intradetrusor botulinum toxin type A in children with neurogenic bladder due to myelomeningocele. J Urol 2006;175(3 Pt 1):1102–5.
65. Kajbafzadeh AM, Moosavi S, Tajik P, et al. Intravesical injection of botulinum toxin type A: management of neuropathic bladder and bowel dysfunction in children with myelomeningocele. Urology 2006;68 (5):1091–6 [discussion: 1096–97].
66. Riccabona M, Koen M, Schindler M, et al. Botulinum-A toxin injection into the detrusor: a safe alternative in the treatment of children with myelomeningocele with detrusor hyperreflexia. J Urol 2004;171(2 Pt 1):845–8 [discussion: 848].
67. Schulte-Baukloh H, Knispel HH, Stolze T, et al. Repeated botulinum-A toxin injections in treatment of children with neurogenic detrusor overactivity. Urology 2005;66(4):865–70 [discussion: 870].
68. Schulte-Baukloh H, Michael T, Schobert J, et al. Efficacy of botulinum-a toxin in children with detrusor hyperreflexia due to myelomeningocele: preliminary results. Urology 2002;59(3):325–7 [discussion: 327–8].
69. Schulte-Baukloh H, Michael T, Sturzebecher B, et al. Botulinum-A toxin detrusor injection as a novel approach in the treatment of bladder spasticity in children with neurogenic bladder. Eur Urol 2003;44(1): 139–43.
70. Game X, Mouracade P, Chartier-Kastler E, et al. Botulinum toxin-A (Botox) intradetrusor injections in children with neurogenic detrusor overactivity/ neurogenic overactive bladder: a systematic literature review. J Pediatr Urol 2009;5(3):156–64.
71. Schurch B, Schmid DM, Stohrer M. Treatment of neurogenic incontinence with botulinum toxin A. N Engl J Med 2000;342(9):665.
72. Ahmed HU, Shergill IS, Arya M, et al. Management of detrusor-external sphincter dyssynergia. Nat Clin Pract Urol 2006;3(7):368–80.
73. Lai HH, Smith CP. Hitting below the belt (bladder): botulinum treatment of urethral and prostate disorders. Curr Urol Rep 2007;8(5):351–8.
74. Dykstra DD, Sidi AA. Treatment of detrusor-sphincter dyssynergia with botulinum A toxin: a double-blind study. Arch Phys Med Rehabil 1990;71(1):24–6.
75. Gallien P, Reymann JM, Amarenco G, et al. Placebo controlled, randomised, double blind study of the effects of botulinum A toxin on detrusor sphincter dyssynergia in multiple sclerosis patients. J Neurol Neurosurg Psychiatr 2005;76(12):1670–6.
76. Kuo HC. Recovery of detrusor function after urethral botulinum A toxin injection in patients with idiopathic low detrusor contractility and voiding dysfunction. Urology 2007;69(1):57–61 [discussion: 61–2].
77. Chuang YC, Yoshimura N, Huang CC, et al. Intravesical botulinum toxin a administration produces analgesia against acetic acid induced bladder pain responses in rats. J Urol 2004;172(4 Pt 1): 1529–32.
78. Abbott JA, Jarvis SK, Lyons SD, et al. Botulinum toxin type A for chronic pain and pelvic floor spasm in women: a randomized controlled trial. Obstet Gynecol 2006;108(4):915–23.
79. Maria G, Brisinda G, Civello IM, et al. Relief by botulinum toxin of voiding dysfunction due to benign prostatic hyperplasia: results of a randomized, placebo-controlled study. Urology 2003;62(2): 259–64 [discussion: 264–5].
80. Zermann D, Ishigooka M, Schubert J, et al. Perisphincteric injection of botulinum toxin type A. A treatment option for patients with chronic prostatic pain? Eur Urol 2000;38(4):393–9.
81. Smith CP, O'Leary M, Erickson J, et al. Botulinum toxin urethral sphincter injection resolves urinary retention after pubovaginal sling operation. Int Urogynecol J Pelvic Floor Dysfunct 2002;13(1):55–6.
82. Khera M, Boone TB, Smith CP. Botulinum toxin type A: a novel approach to the treatment of recurrent urethral strictures. J Urol 2004;172(2):574–5.

The Neurogenic Bladder and Incontinent Urinary Diversion

O. Lenaine Westney, MD

KEYWORDS

• Neurogenic bladder • Ileovesicostomy • Bladder neck
• Incontinence • Urinary stoma

The development of an algorithm for the safe management of the neurogenic bladder has been pivotal in the prevention of urinary tract complications, which previously resulted in high morbidity and mortality in the population with this condition.[1] The introduction of intermittent catheterization by Lapides and colleagues[2] in 1971 furnished the cornerstone of the long-term treatment in patients with neurogenic bladder.[2] Next, the discovery by McGuire and colleagues[3] that storage and leak point pressures greater than 40 cm H_2O were deleterious to the upper tract established a guideline for evaluating the results from urodynamic monitoring and supplied a trigger for management changes in the individual patient. Also, the addition of anticholinergic medical therapy to the treatment armamentarium was an indispensable adjunct to controlling uninhibited detrusor contractions, maintaining storage volumes, and preventing the development of poor compliance.[4,5] The pathophysiology of the neurogenic bladder and the associated urodynamic findings are detailed in the article by McGuire elsewhere in this issue.

Uncontrolled leakage secondary to severe intrinsic sphincter deficiency, detrusor hyperreflexia, or progressively poor compliance can result in a hygiene problem that is difficult to manage in the incapacitated adult patient with neurogenic bladder. A wet perineum can adversely affect attempts to maintain skin integrity and interfere with the ability to treat and heal decubiti. In an effort to achieve a dry perineum, catheter drainage using urethral or suprapubic catheters has been used. However, long-term experience with catheter drainage has demonstrated a wide range of lower and upper tract complications, including urethral erosion, urethrocutaneous fistula, urinary tract infection, development of poor compliance, bladder and upper tract calculi, hydronephrosis, and increased risk of malignancy.[6–9]

CATHETER DRAINAGE: URETHRAL, SUPRAPUBIC, AND CONDOM

In the male patient, the option of external condom drainage exists, assuming that mechanical or functional obstruction is not present at any point from the bladder neck to the urethral meatus. If urethral stricture is present, it must be corrected via urethrotomy or urethroplasty, if necessary. The presence of detrusor sphincter dyssynergia (DSD) has been most commonly treated with either sphincterotomy or urethral stents. Although initially effective, sphincterotomy has been associated with hemorrhage, erectile dysfunction, and the need for retreatment to maintain a low-pressure outlet.[10,11] Urethral stents have compared favorably with sphincterotomy when evaluated in a randomized fashion, with respect to maintenance of low detrusor leak point pressures and residual volumes.[12] Despite the functional success, patients may suffer from pain and dysreflexia. In addition, technical issues may lead to the need for immediate removal, secondary to misplacement or migration, the necessity for placement of an overlapping stent, or stent

Department of Urology, MD Anderson Cancer Center, 1515 Holcombe Boulevard, Unit 1373, Houston, TX 77030, USA
E-mail address: owestney@mdanderson.org

Urol Clin N Am 37 (2010) 581–592
doi:10.1016/j.ucl.2010.07.003

encrustation over time.[13] Alternatively, transurethral or transperineal injection of botulinum toxin A has been demonstrated to be effective in reducing bladder storage pressures, residuals, and external sphincter tone.[14] Similar to mechanical methods for counteracting the sphincter, injection also requires serial evaluations and repetitions.

In the female patient, the option of decreasing outlet resistance for low-pressure drainage is not viable because of the lack of an effective collection device. Therefore, in these situations, the use of a urethral catheter often results in a progressively dilated outlet, which eventually is not sufficiently competent to hold a balloon. At that juncture, change to a suprapubic catheter is ineffective because of continued leakage via the irreversibly damaged bladder neck.

Although clean intermittent catheterization is the mainstay of neurogenic bladder management, in patients with poor manual dexterity, mental deficits, or quadriplegia, reliable ancillary support from family or caretakers is required. Often, this support is not available creating the need for options that offer tubeless, low-pressure drainage without the need for intermittent catheterization; the primary contemporary alternatives are vesicostomy, ileal conduit, or ileovesicostomy. In this context, cutaneous ureterostomy is discussed briefly for historical interest.

CUTANEOUS URETEROSTOMY

Cutaneous ureterostomy was described by Johnston[15] for use in cases of pediatric congenital ureteral or detrusor dysfunction. The ureters were tunneled in an extraperitoneal fashion to the bilateral abdominal or flank stomas or a single stoma, requiring translocation of 1 ureter or ureteroureterostomy. The primary drawbacks of the procedure have been stomal stenosis requiring intubation and pyelonephritis. Contemporary techniques have been introduced to reduce stomal stenosis.[16] Kim and collegues[17] reported on the Toyoda technique, wide spatulation of the ureter combined with skin excision, combined with 4-quadrant fixation of the anterior and posterior rectus sheaths encircling the stoma. With the combined procedure, the resultant catheter-free rate in patients was 90%. However, these patients still experienced high rates of pyelonephritis of 19.4% and 17.4% in the early and late postoperative periods, respectively. Utilization of this technique has been supplanted primarily by the advent of intermittent catheterization and vesicostomy in the pediatric population and endoscopic and percutaneous tube placement in the critically ill or end-stage obstructed patients. However, cutaneous ureterostomy may play a more active role in neurogenic bladder management in developing countries where catheters are less readily available.[18]

VESICOSTOMY

Blocksom[19] is credited with the initial description of the formation of a surgical vesicocutaneous fistula in an adult patient as a tubeless alternative to the suprapubic catheter.[19] The technique was further modified by Lapides and colleagues[20] in 1960 with the use of skin and bladder flaps. Vesicostomy has been most effectively used as a form of incontinent diversion in the pediatric neurogenic population. Low-pressure bladder drainage to a diaper is continued until circumstances permit the initiation of intermittent catheterization (urethral or catheterizable channel), with or without augmentation cystoplasty. However, vesicostomy has also been demonstrated to be an effective form of long-term decompression in a subset of patients who do not have the individual ability or social support to comply with the care associated with continence.[21]

Technique

The technique has varied minimally since its initial description. However, the Duckett modification of the Blocksom technique is designed to decrease the occurrence of stomal-related complications, stenosis and prolapse.[21,22]

A 2-cm midline transverse incision is made midway between the symphysis and lower edge of the umbilicus. A transverse rectus fascia incision exposes the midline of the rectus muscle. A triangular piece of rectus fascia is excised to accommodate a 24F catheter. The bladder is distended to assist in the identification of the detrusor. The perivesical fascia is incised to expose the detrusor. Traction sutures are placed on either side of the planned cystotomy. The dissection is performed extraperitoneally, with the anterior surface of the bladder exposed using traction sutures. Blunt dissection is used to mobilize the bladder further into the incision. The umbilical vessels and urachal remnant are identified and ligated. The urachus and a small portion of the bladder dome are excised. The detrusor is sutured to the fascia circumferentially 1 cm from the lower edge of the cystostomy. The bladder mucosa is everted and sutured to the skin using interrupted sutures.

Duckett[22] emphasizes the proper placement of the stoma to avoid the development of complications. Insufficient mobilization of the bladder surrounding the dome or placement of the stoma too close to the symphysis can lead to prolapse or obstruction, respectively.

Complications

In the absence of an acute obstruction of the stoma caused by an insufficient aperture in the fascia, the remaining complications are long term. Prolapse or stenosis may require surgical revision. In the short term, stenosis can be managed by intermittent catheterization. Bladder calculi must be removed, and stasis corrected if present.

ILEAL CONDUIT

History

The ileal conduit was initially described by Seifert in 1935 and popularized by Bricker in 1950.[23] This technique has been the gold standard for urinary diversion in patients with muscle invasive bladder cancer, against which neobladders and catheterizable diversions are compared.[24] Soon after the introduction of the ileal conduit, the procedure was applied to the population with neurogenic bladder as a mechanism for treating incontinence and counteracting the effects of the poorly compliant bladder on the upper tract.[25–27] In the decades that followed, the larger reported series focused on the use of the conduit in the pediatric population, primarily with spina bifida.[28] This form of management was abandoned because of complications, including progressive renal deterioration (16%–61%), pyocystitis (1%–14%), ureteroileal anastomotic stricture (3%–20%), upper tract calculi (1%–11%), and stomal stenosis (6%–48%).[29] As reported by Elder and colleagues,[30] alteration of the technique to a colonic conduit with an antirefluxing ureteral anastomosis did not change the high level of renal deterioration. Therefore, in the late seventies, management of neurogenic bladder in the pediatric population using the ileal conduit was abandoned in favor of intermittent catheterization and ureteral reimplantation for renal units with reflux. In adult patients, although renal deterioration is a documented long-term complication from ileal conduit diversion, it is less concerning than in the developing pediatric kidney.

Technique

The ileal loop procedure has been essentially unchanged since its introduction, with the exception of a minor modification for the purpose of eliminating complications related to loop redundancy or the stoma. The following is a modified version of the technique from a prior edition of this review series.[31]

A vertical midline incision is performed from the symphysis pubis to the umbilicus. After entering the abdomen, a self-retaining retractor is positioned. The ureters are identified and ligated as distally as possible. Temporarily obstructing the ureter with a tie or clip allows for dilation until it is time for the ureteroileal anastomosis. The ureters are dissected superiorly to the pelvic brim while preserving the adventitia. Starting approximately 15 cm from the ileocecal valve, the distal margin of the proposed ileal segment begins. The length required should be sufficient to span the distance from the stoma site to the sacral promontory. Before deciding on the final limits of the segment, the associated vascular arcades are inspected to ensure that at least 2 vascular arcades are present. Mesenteric windows are formed by dividing the peritoneum, fat, and intervening blood vessels. This division can be performed using mosquito hemostats and ties, a stapler, or the monopolar cautery combined with the LigaSure device (Covidien, Boulder, CO, USA). After manually milking any bowel contents out of the planned segment, the bowel is transected with a 55 mm linear cutter. Bowel continuity is performed using a combination of a 75 mm linear cutter and 60 mm linear stapler or a hand-sewn 2-layer closure. The mesenteric defect is approximated with interrupted 4-0 silk sutures.

The left ureter is passed under the sigmoid colon, superior to the inferior mesenteric artery. Alternatively, the left ureter is brought through the sigmoid colon mesentery. With the proximal end of the loop positioned at the level of the sacral promontory, the ureteroileal anastomosis is performed in a standard end-to-side fashion after ureteral spatulation. Absorbable 4-0 or 5-0 sutures should be used, and suturing may be in an interrupted or running fashion. The remaining step is the formation of the stoma. The plunger of a 10-mL syringe may be used as a guide for the stoma site. The skin followed by subcutaneous tissue and fat is cored out using the monopolar cautery. The fascia is scored in a cruciate manner. Four-quadrant 2-0 absorbable sutures are placed at the points of the fascial incision. The underlying muscle is spread manually, and the peritoneum is punctured through bluntly or scored with the cautery, if necessary. The resulting defect should be sufficient to easily accommodate 2 fingers. A Dennis bowel clamp is passed through the stoma site into the abdomen, and the distal end of the conduit is secured and guided through the abdominal wall. The mesentery should be facing medially. The preplaced fascial sutures are placed through the bowel serosa and tied. The mucosa is everted by suturing from the skin edge, to the serosa at the level of the skin edge, and then to the mucosa and tying with the mucosa folding over the skin border.

Complications: Early and Late

In large series of cystectomy and ileal diversion, the most common short-term complications are ileus, acute pyelonephritis, bowel obstruction, urine leak, and ureteral obstruction. With respect to long-term complications, stomal stenosis, pyelonephritis, metabolic acidosis, and ureteral obstruction are seen most commonly. The primary long-term complications of ileal conduit diversion are centered on stomal/peristomal problems (stomal/peristomal lesions, stomal stenosis, stomal retraction), parastomal hernia, conduit stenosis, and renal deterioration.[24] Overall, complications occur in roughly 60% of patients, and the number of complications increases with the duration of follow-up, making continued surveillance of these patients mandatory.[32]

Complications in the Adult Population with Neurogenic Bladder

Chartier-Kastler and colleagues[33] reported on 33 patients with neurogenic bladder secondary to spinal cord injury or debilitating conditions who underwent ileal conduit with or without cystectomy at a mean follow-up of 48 months. Overall, 12 patients (36%) experienced 18 complications. The early complications were characterized by one incident each of sepsis, acute pyelonephritis, ureteroileal anastomotic leak, pelvic hematoma, and lower extremity thrombophlebitis. In comparison, the most common late complications were pyocystis and pyelonephritis. Of the 19 patients with native bladder, 4 (3 men, 1 woman) experienced pyocystis, resulting in 3 secondary cystectomies. There were no stomal complications reported. In contrast, a series by Singh and colleagues[34] evaluating 93 patients with benign disease (76% neurogenic), at least 2 years after ileal conduit, demonstrated a stomal complication rate of 31%, although most were managed with conservative measures.

Simultaneous Cystectomy

One of the primary decisions to be made when using the ileal conduit for the population with neurogenic bladder is whether cystectomy must be performed at the time of the diversion. The addition of cystectomy adds considerable time and morbidity to the procedure. However, the development of pyocystitis, if not effectively managed conservatively, results in the need for a secondary cystectomy. Chartier-Kastler and colleagues[33] reported that pyocystitis occurred in 21% of patients who did not undergo cystectomy at the time of ileal diversion. Similarly, Singh and colleagues[34] reported that in their series of supravesical diversions, 48 of 93 patients (52%) suffered from pyocystitis and recurrent vesical infections, resulting in the need for 5 delayed cystectomies.[33] Patients who were able to forego cystectomy were managed by scheduled bladder irrigation with solutions containing antimicrobials. In addition, in female patients, creation of an artificial vesicovaginal fistula to allow for drainage of the bladder secretions is an option.[35] Even in consideration of the additional morbidity, for patients who are unable to catheterize or are without social support, serious consideration should be given to concomitant cystectomy.

ILEOVESICOSTOMY

The ileovesicostomy combines the bowel harvest and gastrointestinal tract reconstitution techniques of the ileal conduit without requiring cystectomy or dissection of the ureters. The ileal segment functions as a conduit between the native bladder and the skin. The advantages of the general ease of stoma care are gained while maintaining the native ureterovesical junction, therefore eliminating the complications related to the ureteroileal anastomotic stricture. In addition, the ileovesicostomy can be reversed under the appropriate circumstances for patients who regain the ability to perform urethral catheterization.

History

The basis for the current ileovesicostomy technique originates from the canine experiments of Smith and Hinman[36] in 1955. The investigators described anastomosing the ileum to the native bladder. Therefore, the native bladder would serve as a continent reservoir with preferential low-pressure drainage through the ileal conduit instead of the urethra. This technique was based on the hypothesis that the intact bladder neck would remain functional with voiding initiated by the detrusor contraction. However, in humans with neurogenic bladder, the pressure source would be furnished by uninhibited bladder contractions or the intra-abdominal pressure. A similar technique was translated to children with spina bifida by Cordonnier[37] in 1957. The investigator described a case series of 3 patients in whom he connected a peristaltic ileal segment to the bladder, with the distal end attached to the skin.

Patient Selection

The ideal patient for ileovesicostomy is characterized by the following: (1) an inability or unwillingness to perform intermittent catheterization, (2) a hyperreflexic detrusor, and (3) a small-capacity bladder. Patients with hypocontractile or atonic bladders with or without high capacity are at an increased risk for elevated storage volumes, which may predispose them to recurrent urinary tract infections and/or formation of calculi. Although, these patients may be offered the procedure, long-term management must be tailored to prevent related complications.[38]

Technique: Open

The contemporary ileovesicostomy technique stems from the description by Schwartz and colleagues[39] in 1994. In subsequent patient series' by other investigators, there were minor deviations related to the type of bladder incision, such as wide transverse cystostomy in lieu of the U-shaped flap.[40,41] Regardless of these differences, the surgical principles are based on achieving dependent drainage via a wide ileovesical anastomosis, a judicious selection of conduit length to prevent redundancy, a sufficient aperture in the rectus fascia to prevent future obstruction, and the creation of a stoma conducive to easy appliance fit. The surgical technique as reported by Schwartz and colleagues is depicted in **Fig. 1**.

All patients underwent routine mechanical bowel preparation. The proposed stoma site is marked preoperatively with the aid of an enterostomal therapist. With the patient in the supine or extended lithotomy position the peritoneal cavity is entered through a midline or Gibson incision. The bladder and terminal ileum were exposed, and a posteriorly based wide u-shaped flap was created. A suitable segment of ileum measuring 10 to 15 cm proximal to the ileocecal valve is selected taking care that the isolated segment incorporates 1 or 2 distinct vascular arcades. The segment should be just long enough to reach from the bladder to the pre-marked skin site without redundancy; usually 10 to 15 cm are adequate.

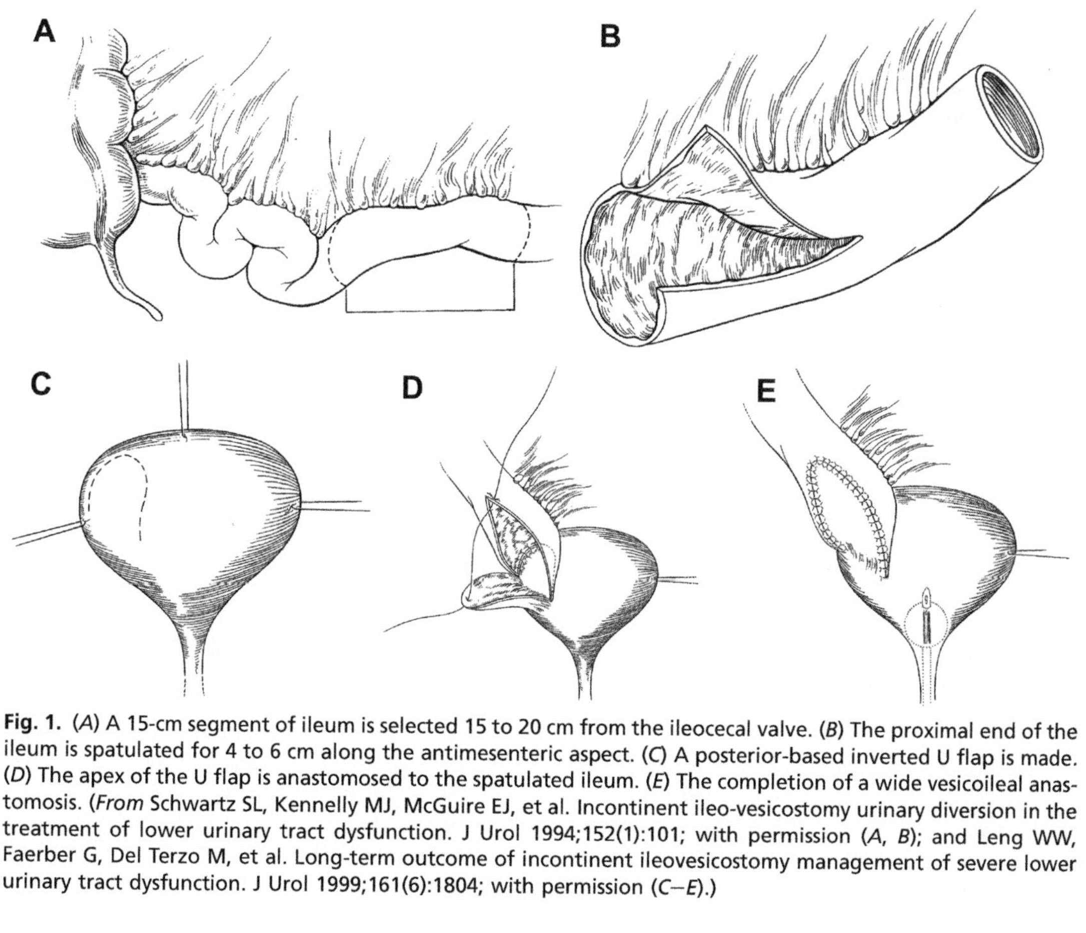

Fig. 1. (*A*) A 15-cm segment of ileum is selected 15 to 20 cm from the ileocecal valve. (*B*) The proximal end of the ileum is spatulated for 4 to 6 cm along the antimesenteric aspect. (*C*) A posterior-based inverted U flap is made. (*D*) The apex of the U flap is anastomosed to the spatulated ileum. (*E*) The completion of a wide vesicoileal anastomosis. (*From* Schwartz SL, Kennelly MJ, McGuire EJ, et al. Incontinent ileo-vesicostomy urinary diversion in the treatment of lower urinary tract dysfunction. J Urol 1994;152(1):101; with permission (*A*, *B*); and Leng WW, Faerber G, Del Terzo M, et al. Long-term outcome of incontinent ileovesicostomy management of severe lower urinary tract dysfunction. J Urol 1999;161(6):1804; with permission (*C–E*).)

The ileum is spatulated by making a 4 to 6 cm incision along the antimesenteric border of the proximal portion. The distal segment is brought through the abdominal wall to the predetermined skin site and a nipple is creased. The proximal ileal segment is anastomosed to the bladder starting posteriorly with a single layer of absorbable suture. A 22F multi-hole catheter is placed through the ileal segment into the bladder before the closure of the anastomosis. Standard urethral closure, if required is accomplished via a transvesical or transvaginal approach in female patients, in whom it is done at the internal meatus. In male patients the urethra is closed, when required at the pelvic diaphragm via a perineal approach.[39]

Minimally Invasive Approaches

Considering the additional challenges in the recovery of a patient with neurogenic bladder from an abdominal incision, theoretically, minimally invasive surgery should have advantages with respect to blood loss, length of hospital stay, and resumption of normal routine.

Laparoscopic approach

There are 2 case reports of ileovesicostomy performed laparoscopically, which demonstrated a similar operative length, decreased blood loss, and shorter length of stay as that of the open series.[42,43] There are no long-term large series reporting the improvement of surgical time or long-term patient outcomes. The key points of the laparoscopic technique reported by Hsu and colleagues[42] are as follows:

1. A 5-port transperitoneal approach with pneumoperitoneum is established using the Hassan technique.
2. The bladder is filled with saline followed by anterior and lateral laparoscopic dissection.
3. Laparoscopic electrocautery scissors are used to create an inverted U cystostomy.
4. The distal end of the planned ileal segment is brought through the infraumbilical port site. Division of the mesentery, harvest of the segment, and restoration of bowel continuity are performed extracorporeally.
5. The proximal staple line is removed. After irrigation, 2 cm of spatulation in the antimesenteric aspect is performed.
6. The bowel is transferred into the abdomen and pneumoperitoneum is reestablished.
7. In preparation for the anastomosis, the proximal end of the ileal segment and U flap are oriented appropriately.
8. Using laparoscopic freehand suturing and intracorporeal knot tying, a single-layer running anastomosis is performed with 2-0 polyglactin.
9. The anastomosis is tested by distending the bladder and attached ileal segment with saline via the urethral Foley catheter.
10. The distal end of the ileum is brought through the right 5-mm port, and the stoma is created.
11. The abdomen is drained with a Jackson-Pratt drain placed via the left 10-mm port site.

In the case report from Abrahams and colleagues,[43] the ileovesicostomy was performed completely intracorporeally. However, the ileum was not spatulated, and the cystostomy corresponded in size. The long-term outcome of this variation in technique has not been reported.

Robotic approach

The advent of minimally invasive robotic devices has resulted in the attempt to use this technology for reconstructive procedures. The benefits of using robotic techniques with respect to decreased blood loss and decreased length of stay has been demonstrated for other urologic procedures and in other surgical disciplines.[44–47] The robot-assisted ileovesicostomy technique has been described by Vanni and colleagues.[48] In general, the robotic approach is similar to the laparoscopic procedure described earlier. The primary differences are as follows:

1. After positioning and establishing pneumoperitoneum to 12 mm Hg, the trocars are placed and the robot is docked.
2. The bladder is distended, and the peritoneum covering the posterior bladder wall is excised.
3. Electrocautery is used to develop a posterior U flap of the following dimensions: 8 cm across at the base, tapering to 3 cm at the tip, and 5 cm long.
4. Preparation of the isolation of a 15-cm ileal segment, including mesenteric window creation, bowel division, and spatulation, is performed intracorporeally.
5. The distal end of the loop is tagged with a 15-cm 3-0 undyed absorbable suture and pulled through the planned stoma site with a Carter-Thompson needle. Sufficient tension is created to retract the conduit during the vesicoenteric anastomosis.
6. The vesicoenteric anastomosis is initiated by securing the mesenteric border of the proximal conduit's proximal enterotomy to the base of the cystotomy with an interrupted absorbable 2-0 polyglactin suture. Then full-thickness running sutures are started at the

6-o'clock position on either side of the anastomosis to the 3-o'clock and 9-o'clock positions on the cystotomy.

7. The anastomosis is completed with the approximation of the U-shaped bladder flap to the spatulated antimesenteric aspect of the ileum.
8. The ends of the native small bowel are tacked together with a dyed suture, which is brought out through the stoma site with a Carter-Thompson needle.
9. Hemostasis maneuvers are performed, the abdomen is irrigated, trocars are removed, and the pneumoperitoneum is released.
10. After creating a 5-cm circumference defect to the level of the rectus fascia at the premarked stoma site, the rectus fascia is incised and the rectus muscles blunt spread to accommodate 2 fingers.
11. On entrance to the peritoneal cavity, the dyed suture is grasped and the native bowel ends are delivered thorough the stomal incision. Bowel continuity is restored extracorporeally with a standard stapled anastomosis and returned to the abdomen.
12. An everting stoma is fashioned with the distal end of the ileal segment.
13. Silastic catheters (16F) are placed per urethra, and the ileal limb is attached to the bladder.

Management of the Outlet

In the patient with associated intrinsic sphincter deficiency, it is necessary to make a decision whether to close the bladder neck or increase the outlet resistance at that level with a sling, pubovaginal or perineal. Patients with stricture disease or DSD have an existing barrier to urethral leakage. The problem of the incontinent outlet is magnified in female patients with a grossly dilated bladder neck and urethra secondary to urethral catheter erosion. In patients with a urethral leak point pressure less than what is commonly achieved on average via the ileovesicostomy stoma (<10 cm H_2O), it would be mandatory to address the outlet simultaneously with ileovesicostomy.[49] With regard to selecting bladder neck closure versus pubovaginal sling, Tan and colleagues[50] reported higher postoperative complication rates in patients who underwent concomitant placement of a sling.

Bladder neck closure can be complicated by the development of vesicourethral fistula in the adult and pediatric populations.[51–54] An additional challenge in the adult population is the common unavailability of omentum because of prior multiple surgical procedures. Stoffel and McGuire[55] reported on 18 patients who underwent bladder neck closure with a final continence rate of 88%. However, 5 patients underwent an average of 3.8 additional surgeries to achieve continence. There are multiple reports of different techniques aimed at improving the success of bladder neck closure, including flap interposition using omental, Martius, and vascularized pedicle flaps.[56] Persistent or recurrent incontinence despite multiple attempts at bladder neck closure may result in the need for delayed cystectomy and conversion of the ileovesicostomy limb to an ileal conduit.

Postoperative Care

Cystography is performed 2 to 3 weeks after surgery to ensure a watertight reservoir anastomosis. An important element of postoperative care includes the patient/caregiver instruction in routine irrigation of the ileovesicostomy to prevent mucous plugging and any nidus of infection. It is prudent to perform a serial evaluation of the patient who has undergone ileovesicostomy in the form of yearly cystometric assessment of detrusor leak point pressure and ultrasonography of the upper urinary tract. In patients who report problems, such as febrile urinary tract infection, bladder pain, or hematuria, comprehensive testing in the form of video urodynamics, cystoscopy, and/or urine cytology is indicated. From a surveillance standpoint, cystoscopy should be performed either through the urethra or stoma, starting 3 to 5 years after ileovesicostomy because of the risk of bladder cancer.[50]

Complications: Early and Late

Early

Early postoperative complications are not consistently reported in all ileovesicostomy series. However, with the exception of complications directly related to the ileovesicostomy and/or bladder neck closure, such as immediate limb/stomal obstruction and perineal leakage, the remainder are consistent with major abdominal surgery, such as wound infection, wound dehiscence, small bowel obstruction/ileus, and sepsis.[38,50]

Management of Late Complications

Ileovesicostomy limb outlet obstruction

Obstruction of the ileal limb can occur by one or a combination of 4 mechanisms: (1) ileovesicostomy anastomotic stricture, (2) ileal limb kink, (3) extrinsic compression by fascial stenosis, and (4) stomal stenosis (**Table 1**). The presence of one of these mechanical problems may be heralded by poor drainage, urethral leakage, stone

Table 1
Long-term ileovesicostomy complications

References	Number of Patients	Follow-up (mo)	Recurrent Urinary Tract Infection	Bladder Stones	Upper Tract Stones	Urethral Incontinence	Fascial/ Stomal Stenosis	Revision to Ileal Conduit	Delayed Bladder Neck Closure
Mutchnik et al[40] (1997)	6	13.1	1 (16)	0	0	1 (16)	0	0	1 (16)
Atan et al[63] (1999)	15	23.2	3 (20)	3 (20)	5 (33)	4 (25)	2 (13)	1 (7)	—
Gudziak et al[62] (1999)	13	23	1 (8)	0	1 (8)	1 (8)	1 (8)	0	—
Leng et al[49] (1999)	38	52	1 (3)	2 (5)	4 (10)	—	2 (5)	—	—
Gauthier and Winters[41] (2003)	7	37.4	1 (14)	0	1 (14)	0	1 (14)	—	—
Tan et al[50] (2008)	50	26.3	—	3 (6)	1 (2)	—	14 (28)	0	13 (26)
Zimmerman and Santucci[38] (2009)	8	—	—	—	—	1	—	—	2
Hellenthal et al[57] (2009)	12	66	8 (66)	1 (8)	1 (8)	1 (8)	2 (16)	2 (16)	0

formation, or recurrent urinary tract infection. Stenosis at the level of the skin may be suggested on examination. More proximal obstruction can be identified by the inability to introduce a finger into the stoma past the fascial level or by difficulty in catheterization. The passage of a catheter into the bladder yielding a residual of greater than 100 mL in the hyperreflexic bladder is reflective of obstruction. The most functional and definitive test is a fluoroscopic urodynamic study, with the sensor filling via the urethra if possible. Obstruction caused by an anastomotic stricture, kink, or stenosis can be clearly identified along with the detrusor leak point pressure. Cystoscopic evaluation of the limb is a useful visual correlate to the radiologic appearance.[49]

All mechanical issues related to obstruction or limb redundancy require surgical intervention for definitive management. However, the limb can be catheterized intermittently for short-term management to ensure appropriate drainage until surgical revision can be performed.

Incontinence

On the complaint of continued or recurrent perineal leakage, the source must be clearly identified. In the case of patients who underwent simultaneous bladder neck or urethral closure, it must be determined whether urine is passing via a recanalization between the bladder and urethra or the formation of a new fistula between the bladder and vagina or perineum. In the report by Stoffel and McGuire,[55] the mean time to failure after initial bladder neck closure is 1 month. Identification of the tract may require infusion of contrast through the ileovesicostomy via an inflated Foley catheter. Cystoscopic evaluation is also necessary in assessing the location and size of the fistula. Depending on the quality of the perineal and adjacent tissue, interposition of a vascularized pedicle flap may be necessary in addition to closure. Failure to maintain closure of the urethra is the most common indication to switch to cystectomy and ileal conduit.

Urethral incontinence in patients with the open bladder neck may be an indication of limb obstruction at any location from the vesicoileal anastomosis to the stoma.

Febrile urinary tract infection/urosepsis

Recurrent or febrile urinary tract infection may signal a mechanical problem caused by ileal limb obstruction. This diagnosis is best documented urodynamically and in most cases requires surgical intervention. In situations in which no mechanical cause can be identified, it may be necessary to use prophylactic antimicrobial therapy or bladder irrigation.[57]

Upper tract calculi/bladder calculi

Even in the absence of urinary diversion, patients with spinal cord injury are at a higher risk of developing urinary tract calculi.[58,59] After evaluation to ensure that the cause of the calculus formation is not related to the improper functioning of the ileal limb, upper and lower tract calculi should be managed based on treatment guidelines. However, there must be meticulous attention to patient positioning and preoperative urine culture to assure appropriate perioperative antibiotic selection.[60,61] In patients who have not undergone closure of the bladder neck, access to the bladder may be gained via the ileovesicostomy limb.

Urodynamic outcomes: leak point pressure

The primary goal of ileovesicostomy is the creation of low-pressure drainage ideally with low storage volumes or residuals in the bladder. Not all series furnish the preoperative and/or postoperative leak point pressures; however, those with these data are detailed in **Table 2**.[40,41,62,63] Most of the remaining series confirm the resolution of hydronephrosis, maintenance of renal function, and/or no development of new vesicoureteral reflux.

Table 2
Preoperative and postoperative leak point pressure data

References	Number of Patients	Mean Follow-up (mo)	Preoperative Leak Point Pressure (Mean cm H_2O)	Postoperative Leak Point Pressure (Mean cm H_2O)
Mutchnik et al[40] (1997)	6	13.1	40.1	7.7
Atan et al[63] (1999)	15	23.2	—	—
Gudziak et al[62] (1999)	13	23	—	8.2
Gauthier and Winters[41] (2003)	7	37.4	42.7	16.7

SUMMARY

Low-pressure drainage without the use of indwelling catheters characterizes the ideal technique in long-term management of the neurogenic bladder. Patients who lack the desire or physical/mental capability to perform intermittent catheterization may require surgical reconstruction to achieve tubeless incontinence drainage via a controlled stoma. Cutaneous ureterostomy is no longer an actively used form of primary management of the neurogenic bladder. The vesicostomy is an effective mechanism for low-pressure drainage but is predominantly used in the pediatric population as a temporizing measure. Ileal conduit, the gold standard for urinary diversion postcystectomy, has been successfully applied to the adult population with neurogenic bladder. The primary management decision is whether cystectomy is necessary for the prevention of pyocystitis in the individual patient. Ileovesicostomy maintains the native bladder and ureterovesical junction. The management issues specific to this procedure relate to perineal urine leakage, urethral or fistulous; lower tract stones; and ileovesical anastomotic stricture. Both ileal conduit and ileovesicostomy procedures are subject to long-term stoma-related complications.

REFERENCES

1. Frankel HL, Coll JR, Charlifue SW, et al. Long-term survival in spinal cord injury: a fifty year investigation. Spinal Cord 1998;36:266–74.
2. Lapides J, Diokno C, Silber SJ, et al. Clean, intermittent self-catheterization in the treatment of urinary tract disease. Trans of the Amer Assoc of GU Surg 1971;63:92–6.
3. McGuire EJ, Woodside JR, Borden TA, et al. Prognostic value of urodynamic testing in myelodysplastic patients. J Urol 1981;126(2):205–9.
4. Stöhrer M, Murtz G, Kramer G, et al. Propiverine compared to oxybutynin in neurogenic detrusor overactivity—results of a randomized, double-blind, multicenter clinical study. Eur Urol 2007;51:235–42.
5. Goessl C, Knispel HH, Fiedler U, et al. Urodynamic effects of oral oxybutynin chloride in children with myelomeningocele and detrusor hyperreflexia. Urology 1998;51:94–8.
6. Larsen LD, Chamberlin DA, Khonsari F, et al. Retrospective analysis of urologic complications in male patients with spinal cord injury managed with and without indwelling urinary catheters. Urology 1997;50:418–22.
7. Ord J, Lunn D, Reynard J. Bladder management and risk of bladder stone formation in spinal cord injured patients. J Urol 2003;170:1734–7.
8. Ku JH, Choi WJ, Lee KY, et al. Complications of the upper urinary tract in patients with spinal cord injury: a long-term follow-up study. Urol Res 2005;33(6):435–9.
9. Ku JH, Jung TY, Lee JK, et al. Risk factors for urinary stone formation in men with spinal cord injury: a 17-year follow-up study. BJU Int 2006;97(4):790–3.
10. Ahmed HU, Shergill IS, Arya M, et al. Management of detrusor-external sphincter dyssynergia. Nat Clin Pract Urol 2006;3(7):368–80.
11. Reynard JM, Vass J, Sullivan ME, et al. Sphincterotomy and the treatment of detrusor sphincter dyssynergia: current status, future prospects. Spinal Cord 2003;41:1–11.
12. Chancellor MB, Bennett C, Simoneau AR, et al. Sphincteric stent versus external sphincterotomy in spinal cord injured men: prospective randomized multicenter study. J Urol 1999;161:1893–8.
13. Gajewski J, Chancellor MB, Ackman CF, et al. Removal of UroLume endoprosthesis: experience of the North American Study Group for Detrusor-Sphincter Dyssynergia Application. J Urol 2000;163:773–6.
14. Leippold T, Reitz A, Schurch B. Botulinum toxin as a new therapy option for voiding disorders: current state of the art. Eur Urol 2003;44(2):165–74.
15. Johnston JH. Temporary cutaneous ureterostomy in the management of advanced congenital urinary obstruction. Arch Dis Child 1963;38:161–6.
16. Toyoda Y. A new technique for catheterless cutaneous ureterostomy. J Urol 1977;117:276–8.
17. Kim CJ, Wakabayashi Y, Sakano Y, et al. Simple technique for improving tubeless cutaneous ureterostomy. Urology 2005;65(6):1221–5.
18. Chitale SV, Chitale VR. Bilateral ureterocutaneostomy with modified stoma: long-term follow-up. World J Urol 2006;24(2):220–3.
19. Blocksom B. Bladder pouch for prolonged tubeless cystostomy. J Urol 1957;78:398–401.
20. Lapides J, Ajemian EP, Lichtwald JR. Cutaneous vesicostomy. J Urol 1960;84:609–14.
21. Hutcheson JC, Cooper CS, Canning DA, et al. The use of vesicostomy as permanent urinary diversion in the child with myelomeningocele. J Urol 2001;166:2351–3.
22. Duckett JW. Cutaneous vesicostomy in childhood. The Blocksom technique. Urol Clin North Am 1974;1(3):485–95.
23. Woodruff MW, Oberheim WS. Urinary diversion in the treatment of the neurogenic bladder. Urol Clin North Am 1974;1(1):99–111.
24. Hautmann RE, Abol-Enein H, Hafez K, et al. Urinary diversion. Urology 2007;69(1):17–49.
25. Clark K. Ileal conduit urinary diversion in adults with acquired neurogenic bladder. J Trauma 1962;2:142–6.

26. Leadbetter WF, Shaffer FG. Ileal loop diversion: its application to the treatment of neurogenic bladder dysfunction. J Urol 1956;75(3):470–9.
27. Straffon RA, Turnbull RB Jr, Mercer RD. The ileal conduit in the management of children with neurogenic lesions of the bladder. J Urol 1963;89: 198–206.
28. Smith ED. Follow-up studies on 150 ileal conduits in children. J Pediatr Surg 1972;7:1–10.
29. Cass AS, Luxenberg M, Gleich P, et al. A 22-year follow-up of ileal conduits in children with neurogenic bladder. J Urol 1984;132:529–31.
30. Elder DD, Moisey CU, Rees RWM. A long-term follow-up of the colonic conduit operation in children. Br J Urol 1979;51:462–5.
31. Williams O, Vereb MJ, Libertino JA. Noncontinent urinary diversion. Urol Clin North Am 1997;24(4): 735–44.
32. Madersbacher S, Schmidt J, Eberle JM, et al. Long-term outcome of ileal conduit diversion. J Urol 2003; 169:985–90.
33. Chartier-Kastler EJ, Mozer P, Denys P, et al. Neurogenic bladder management and cutaneous non-continent ileal conduit. Spinal Cord 2002;40: 443–8.
34. Singh G, Wilkinson JM, Thomas DG. Supravesical diversion for incontinence: a long-term follow-up. Br J Urol 1998;79:348–53.
35. Fazili T, Bhat TR, Masood S, et al. Fate of the leftover bladder after supravesical urinary diversion for benign disease. J Urol 2006;176:620–1.
36. Smith GI, Hinman F Jr. The intussuscepted ileal cystostomy. J Urol 1955;73(2):261–9.
37. Cordonnier JJ. Ileocystostomy for neurogenic bladder. J Urol 1957;78(5):605–10.
38. Zimmerman WB, Santucci RA. Ileovesicostomy update: changes for the 21st century. Adv Urol 2009;1:1–7.
39. Schwartz SL, Kennelly MJ, McGuire EJ, et al. Incontinent ileo-vesicostomy urinary diversion in the treatment of lower urinary tract dysfunction. J Urol 1994; 152(1):99–102.
40. Mutchnik SE, Hinson JL, Nickell KG, et al. Ileovesicostomy as an alternative form of bladder management in tetraplegic patients. Urol 1997;49 (3):353–7.
41. Gauthier R Jr, Winters JC. Incontinent ileovesicostomy in the management of neurogenic bladder dysfunction. Neurourol Urodyn 2003;22(2):142–6.
42. Hsu THS, Rackley RR, Abdelmalak JB, et al. Laparoscopic ileovesicostomy. J Urol 2002;168(1):180–1.
43. Abrahams HM, Rahman NU, Meng MV, et al. Pure laparoscopic ileovesicostomy. J Urol 2003;170(2 Pt 1): 517–8.
44. Wang AJ, Bhayani SB. Robotic partial nephrectomy versus laparoscopic partial nephrectomy for renal cell carcinoma: single-surgeon analysis of >100 consecutive procedures. Urology 2009;73(2): 306–10.
45. Geisler JP, Orr CJ, Khurshid N, et al. Robotically assisted laparoscopic radical hysterectomy compared with open radical hysterectomy. Int J Gynecol Cancer 2010;20(3):438–42.
46. Snyder BE, Wilson T, Leong BY, et al. Robotic-assisted Roux-en-Y gastric bypass: minimizing morbidity and mortality. Obes Surg 2010;20(3):265–70.
47. Geller EJ, Siddiqui NY, Wu JM, et al. Short-term outcomes of robotic sacrocolpopexy compared with abdominal sacrocolpopexy. Obstet Gynecol 2008;112(6):1201–6.
48. Vanni AJ, Cohen MS, Stoffel JT. Robotic-assisted ileovesicostomy: initial results. Urology 2009;74(4): 814–8.
49. Leng WW, Faerber G, Del Terzo M, et al. Long-term outcome of incontinent ileovesicostomy management of severe lower urinary tract dysfunction. J Urol 1999;161(6):1803–6.
50. Tan HJ, Stoffel J, Daignault S, et al. Ileovesicostomy for adults with neurogenic bladders: complications and potential risk factors for adverse outcomes. Neurourol Urodyn 2008;27(3):238–43.
51. Nguyen HT, Baskin LS. The outcome of bladder neck closure in children with severe urinary incontinence. J Urol 2003;169:1114–6.
52. Jayanthi VR, Churchill BM, McLorie GA, et al. Concomitant bladder neck closure and Mitrofanoff diversion for the management of intractable urinary incontinence. J Urol 1995;154:886–8.
53. Andrews HO, Shah PJR. Surgical management of urethral damage in neurologically impaired female patients with chronic indwelling catheters. BJU 1998;82:820–4.
54. Hall J, Thomas DG. Surgical closure of the bulbar urethra for the treatment of intractable urinary incontinence in the paralyzed patient. BJU 1998; 82:912.
55. Stoffel JT, McGuire EJ. Outcome of urethral closure in patients with neurologic impairment and complete urethral destruction. Neurourol Urodyn 2006;25: 19–22.
56. Smith EA, Kaye JD, Lee JY, et al. Use of rectus abdominis muscle flap as adjunct to bladder neck closure in patients with neurogenic incontinence: preliminary experience. J Urol 2010;183:1556–60.
57. Hellenthal NJ, Short SS, O'Connor RC, et al. Incontinent ileovesicostomy: long-term outcomes and complications. Neurourol Urodyn 2009;28:483–6.
58. Chen Y, DeVivo MJ, Roseman JM. Current trend and risk factors for kidney stones in persons with spinal cord injury: a longitudinal study. Spinal Cord 2000; 38:346–53.
59. Kohl A, Lamed S. Risk factors for renal stone formation in patients with spinal cord injury. Br J Urol 1986; 58:588–91.

60. Rubenstein JN, Gonzalez CM, Blunt LW, et al. Safety and efficacy of percutaneous nephrolithotomy in patients with neurogenic bladder dysfunction. Urol 2004;63:636–40.
61. Sot MC, Lee BR. Urolithiasis in patients with spinal cord injuries: risk factors, management, and outcomes. Curr Opin Urol 2006;16(2):93–9.
62. Gudziak MR, Tiguert R, Puri K, et al. Management of neurogenic bladder dysfunction with incontinent ileovesicostomy. Urol 1999;54(6):1008–11.
63. Atan A, Konety BR, Nangia A, et al. Advantages and risks of ileovesicostomy for the management of neuropathic bladder. Urology 1999;54(4): 636–40.

Bladder Tissue Engineering

Irina Stanasel, MD, Majid Mirzazadeh, MD, John J. Smith III, MD*

KEYWORDS

• Tissue engineering • Stem cells • Bladder regeneration

The properly functioning urinary bladder is composed of a compliant muscular wall and highly specialized urothelium. When operating effectively, it provides a low-pressure, high-capacity reservoir while simultaneously protecting the upper urinary tract from pressure, reflux of urine, and infection. Specialized characteristics of the bladder's smooth muscle fibers, nerves, and blood vessels permit repeated coordinated bladder contractions without compromising storage capability or upper tract protection. When this organ becomes damaged, any attempt at replacing it, in whole or part, must take into consideration all these properties, including reproducing or recreating them.

The bladder can lose the ability to store and empty effectively as a result of numerous conditions, such as cancer, trauma, infection, inflammation, or iatrogenic injury. Additionally, congenital or neurologic conditions, such as spina bifida or spinal cord injury, can also cause progressive loss of bladder function resulting in debilitating urinary incontinence or renal impairment. Conservative methods can be used to maximize patient safety and quality of life when there is mild-to-moderate bladder dysfunction, including behavioral training, clean intermittent catheterization, suprapubic catheterization, and pharmaceuticals. However, when conservative measures fail to protect the upper tracts or lead to worsening quality of life, surgical reconstruction of the bladder is usually considered. The present gold standard, augmentation cystoplasty, can be performed with the use of the small bowel, large bowel, or less often, stomach. Autoaugmentation, described as a partial removal of the detrusor while sparing the urothelium, has also been advocated as a solution in subsets of patients. However, the potential complications from the use of a portion of the gastrointestinal tract to perform augmentation cystoplasty are well characterized. They include urinary tract infections, intestinal obstruction, mucus production, electrolyte abnormalities, perforation, and carcinogenesis.[1,2] In many patients with neurogenic bladder, particularly those with spina bifida, surgical reconstruction of the bladder with the bowel can impact fecal transit time, and this risk needs to be reviewed thoroughly with the patient and family. All these issues beg for an alternate solution.

Tissue engineering was proposed as an alternative for generating bladder tissue for reconstruction in the early 1990s, and tremendous progress has been made in this field since that time. Tissue engineering, as defined by Langer and Vacanti in 1993, is "an interdisciplinary field that applies the principles of engineering and life sciences toward the development of biologic substitutes that restore, maintain or improve tissue function or a whole organ."[3] Tissue engineering identifies the body's own potential for regeneration and supports this propensity with appropriate raw materials and growth factors so that the body's original structure and function may be restored. Tissue engineering can involve the use of a scaffold or matrix alone, wherein the body's natural ability to regenerate is primarily used, or the use of cell-seeded matrices, in which regeneration is even further promoted. Both these technologies have been studied in the quest to develop an engineered bladder.

Department of Urology, Wake Forest University School of Medicine, Medical Center Boulevard, Winston-Salem, NC 27157, USA
* Corresponding author.
E-mail address: jjsmith@wfubmc.edu

Urol Clin N Am 37 (2010) 593–599
doi:10.1016/j.ucl.2010.06.008
0094-0143/10/$ – see front matter

The use of unseeded matrices involves in vivo implantation of bioactive or resorbable matrices. The goal of this technology is to allow the body's natural capability to use the matrix as a scaffold for regeneration. Cell-seeded matrices are scaffolds that are seeded in vitro with autologous cells that have been appropriately cultured. The goal of both technologies is to deliver an implant that has the functional characteristics of the human bladder, while carrying a low-safety risk by having low immunogenic and low tumorigenic potential. A study published by Jayo and colleagues[4] reported on the use of cell-seeded and unseeded biodegradable polyglycolic acid scaffolds for large bladder replacement procedures in the canine subtotal cystectomy model. The early stromal and cellular events occurring after implantation were studied in an attempt to determine whether cell-seeded constructs promoted regeneration better than matrices alone. The constructed neobladders of the cell-seeded group demonstrated predominance of myogenic precursors associated with regeneration, whereas the bare matrix tissues demonstrated a predominance of collagen, which is associated with scar formation rather than regeneration. The seeded group outperformed the unseeded group, with resultant bladders having a greater capacity and near-normal bladder compliance. The tissue in the seeded group also appeared more similar to bladder tissue histologically, as it had a urothelial layer, a suburothelial layer, and a smooth muscle layer. The unseeded scaffolds resulted in re-epithelialization of the graft lumen with fibrosis, graft contraction, and small bladder capacity. These findings led to a conclusion that seeded scaffolds are superior to unseeded, particularly when demand for a large portion of bladder tissue exists, because they promote a regenerative process as opposed to a reparative process.

Harvesting cells from the organ of interest and culturing them has become an important tool in tissue engineering. Autologous bladder cells are harvested from the diseased organ, separated into cell lines of interest, and expanded in vitro to sufficient quantities. They can then be seeded onto matrices to create tissue for implantation back into the host. Previous work has demonstrated that in certain populations, such as in patients with a neurogenic bladder, cells can be safely and effectively harvested and cultured. However, the search for cells that possess more characteristics of healthy tissue and have more regenerative potential continues. Smooth muscle cells from neuropathic bladders have shown abnormal growth, less contractile ability, and inferior adherence compared with normal controls, making them less than ideal cells for culture in this particular population.[5] Other sources of cells are also important, because often, the diseased bladder does not contain enough normal cells to begin expansion. The patient's own cells may also not be desirable for creation of new bladder tissue, as is the case in patients with previously demonstrated bladder malignancy. Multiple possibilities for sources of cells have been investigated, including stem cells and differentiated cells from organs other than the bladder; however, to date, autologous bladder cells remain the gold standard for culture and seeding.

ALTERNATIVE SOURCES OF CELLS

Stem cells hold great promise when autologous cells from the bladder cannot be harvested. The 2 characteristics that define stem cells are self-renewal, or the ability to divide and produce identical cells, and potency, the ability to differentiate into specialized cells.[6] Totipotent stem cells that are formed when an egg and sperm merge can differentiate into embryonic and extraembryonic cell types and can construct a complete, viable organism. Stem cells that can differentiate into cells from all 3 germ layers are descendants of totipotent cells and are called pluripotent, whereas the ones that are more restricted are multipotent. The use of stem cells avoids graft rejection and use of long-term medications needed with allogenic transplantation. Much research has been performed in the area of in vitro stem cell differentiation to produce smooth muscle and urothelial derivatives.

Pluripotent stem cells are of great interest in tissue engineering because of their unlimited self-renewal potential and their ability to differentiate into any cell type of endodermal, mesodermal, or ectodermal lineage.[6] The isolation of pluripotent cells, called embryonic cells, from the inner cell mass of the blastocysts of mice was first performed by Evans and Kaugman[7] in 1981. Subsequently, techniques have been developed to direct these cells to differentiate into specific tissue types. Human embryonic stem cells were isolated in 1998 from unused in vitro fertilization embryos.[8] Sixty cell lines were initially developed from these embryos, 21 of which exist today and are viable and approved for funding by the National Institute of Health. Subsequently, other cell lines have also been developed nationally and internationally. Human embryonic stem cells are surrounded by ethical and moral concerns because of the need for destruction of human embryos to develop these cell lines. Their use has prompted a reevaluation of what, in fact, constitutes the beginning of human life, which is beyond the scope of this article.

Two types of nuclear cloning have been described and developed. Further elucidation of their definition could help in the development of guidelines and laws for the use of embryonic cell lines. Reproductive cloning is used to generate an embryo with the identical genetic make up of its source and is banned in most countries. Therapeutic cloning, otherwise called somatic cell nuclear transfer, uses a donor oocyte with its nuclear material removed and replaced with nuclear material from a donor cell. The autologous stem cell lines developed using this technique have the potential to become any type of cell in the adult body.[6] Currently, this technology is still inefficient and limited. The ethical and social issues associated with embryonic stem cells are complex, and guidelines and laws surrounding their use need to be developed if their use is to become clinically widespread. Issues apart from the ethical and legal ones exist, which have halted the routine use of embryonic stem cells. Their ability to proliferate indefinitely is an important reason that embryonic cells are so attractive but also feared, because this uncontrolled proliferation potential could be associated with tumorigenesis and teratoma formation in the recipient.[6]

A new and exciting advancement in stem cell research involves genetic reprogramming. This technique involves the dedifferentiation of adult somatic cells to produce patient-specific pluripotent stem cells or induced pluripotent state cells. This technique was first described in 2006; however, cells were shown to be incompletely reprogrammed in that pilot study.[9] Subsequent studies were performed using human rather than mouse cells and revealed complete reprogramming of cells.[10,11] There being no need for embryos, the ethical and social issues related to embryonic stem cells are avoided.

An alternate source of stem cells is the amniotic fluid and the placenta. Multiple partially differentiated cell types derived from the fetus have been identified in the amniotic fluid and are referred to as amniotic fluid and placental stem cells.[12] They could be obtained via amniocentesis, chorionic villi sampling, or from the placenta at the time of birth. The cells could be banked to provide a source for autologous therapy later in life or for matching of histocompatible donor cells with recipients. These cells express embryonic and adult stem cell markers. They have been shown to retain long telomeres and a normal karyotype for more than 250 population doublings, making them genetically stable. Thus, they lack the teratoma-forming characteristics of embryonic stem cells, although maintaining the ability to differentiate into cells of all 3 embryonic germ layers.[12] However, additional studies must be conducted to better characterize their differentiation potential and their limitations, as well as to characterize their malignancy potential.

Urine has also been investigated as a potential source of cells and would be an attractive option, because it would provide cells for tissue regeneration in a noninvasive manner. Recent studies have isolated cells from adult urine samples with progenitor cell features and the potential to differentiate into several bladder cell lineages, including cells with urothelial, smooth muscle, endothelial, and interstitial cell markers. These urine progenitor cells comprise only 0.2% of urine cells, but these cells that are found in sparse numbers may hold great promise for future tissue regeneration. The cells are easily cultured, appear genetically stable after several passages, and maintain their ability to give rise to more differentiated cells. They express markers, such as c-Kit, SSEA4, and CD44, which are associated with stem cells. The use of these cells also avoids ethical issues, because they are autologous somatic cells; however, their self-renewal potential has not yet been clearly defined.[13]

Adult stem cells are a potential source of smooth muscle cells for bladder tissue engineering. They are particularly attractive, because they avoid the ethical problems associated with embryonic stem cells. However, they are found only in sparse numbers in the host, do not expand well in cultures, and have a more restricted differentiation potential. Adult stem cells have been isolated from bone marrow, skeletal muscle, adipose tissue, lung, testis, umbilical cord, and placenta. Mesenchymal stem cells are found in the bone marrow and have been studied as a source of bladder cells for seeding of matrices. These cells could be especially helpful in engineering bladders for patients with bladder cancer who need bladder augmentation, because the bone marrow is not a target for bladder cancer metastases, making these cells safe for use in this patient population.[14] These cells have been shown to have the capability to differentiate into a large number of cells and the ability to differentiate into various specialized cell types under appropriate conditions. Expansion and differentiation of bone marrow mesenchymal stem cells varies with external signals and with the environment in which they are grown. Recently, bone marrow mesenchymal cells have been shown to be able to differentiate into mesodermal and endodermal cell lines, and a recent study was conducted to determine their potential to differentiate into multiple cell types. This study showed that bone marrow-derived mesenchymal stem cells demonstrated urothelium-specific genes and proteins , including uroplakin-Ia, cytokeratin-7, and cytokeratin-13. The urothelium-derived medium contained several growth factors, including endothelial growth factor, platelet-derived growth factor (PDGF-BB), transforming growth factor (TGF-B1), and vascular endothelial growth factor (VEGF). However, the cells demonstrated smooth muscle cell genes and proteins when cocultured with smooth muscle cells or in a smooth muscle cell medium, specifically desmin and myosin. Several growth factors were detected in this growth medium as well, and included hepatocyte growth factor, PDGF-BB, TGF-B1, and VEGF.[15] Scaffolds have proven useful for expansion of bone-marrow mesenchymal cells. These have included natural small intestine submucosa[16] and synthetic 3-dimensional (3D) nanofibrous scaffolds, such as poly-L-lactic acid polymer.[14] Further studies are needed to evaluate whether these cells are transformed permanently and to characterize the physical properties of the engineered tissue.

SCAFFOLDS

Another critical aspect of regenerating a large portion of bladder tissue is the bioscaffold selection. The scaffold must possess certain mechanical and physical properties to allow the organ to develop into a desired shape and maintain it. Currently, 2 categories of bladder bioscaffold are used in bladder tissue engineering: natural and synthetic matrices. Natural matrices were among the first to be used and they included skin, preserved bladder, omentum, peritoneum, lyophilized dura mater, chemically treated amniotic membrane, and calcium-treated pericardium. Graft rejection, urinary tract infection, and calculus formation are among the problems encountered with the use of natural matrices. The development of decellularized, naturally derived tissue matrices made of collagen and alginate were aimed at minimizing some of the problems encountered with natural tissue matrices. Decellularized small intestine submucosa has been extensively studied as a scaffold for bladder augmentation. The submucosa is harvested from the jejunum of pigs. However, the process of decellularizing the matrices affects their strength and quality and their ability to provide a reliable scaffold for regeneration and remodeling. A study[17] showed that large bladder augmentation with cell-seeded or unseeded small intestinal submucosa matrix did not improve bladder regeneration. The muscle regenerated was disorganized and its vascularization was poor. The bladders had poor compliance, mostly thought to result from the lack of strength of the natural matrix. The matrix collapses rather than maintaining the shape of the organ. Newer research has focused on evaluating ways to make natural collagen scaffolds more effective, because collagen has great potential to be a valuable scaffold because of its good biocompatibility. A recent study focused on applying plastic compression to achieve higher concentrations of collagen, showing the scaffolds to have an increase in the desirable mechanical properties at the neotissue level.[18] However, natural matrices are still liable to maintain a certain amount of cellularity and thus provide immunogenic components to the recipient.

To overcome some of these challenges encountered in the use of natural matrices, synthetic polymers, such as polyglycolic acid (PGA) and polylactic co-glycolic acid, have been developed and used. These polymers provide enough strength to maintain the shape of the organ. They are also porous materials that allow for the exchange of gas and nutrients and thus promote cell metabolism and growth. These synthetic materials are readily available and their properties are malleable.[4]

CLINICAL APPLICATION

The most complete clinical trial for tissue engineering in urology to date was published in 2006.[19] It involved the engineering of human bladder tissue for young patients with end-stage bladder disease by isolating autologous bladder urothelial and muscle cells, expanding the cells, and attaching them to matrices. Seven patients with myelomeningocele who ranged in age from 4 to 19 years participated in this trial. They all had high-pressure, poorly compliant bladders, and were identified as candidates for augmentation cystoplasty. They each underwent a bladder biopsy for harvesting of urothelial and smooth muscle cells, which were then expanded and seeded on a biodegradable, bladder-shaped scaffold. Based on initial preclinical studies, a collaged matrix derived from decellularized bladder submucosa was used for seeding the cells of the first 3 patients without an omental wrap of the implanted tissue. Further animal studies demonstrated that wrapping the implanted tissue in omentum improved vascularization and that collagen PGA composite matrices performed better in the long term. After realizing that omental wrapping was beneficial to the vascularization of the tissue in vivo, the protocol was revised, and one patient underwent implantation with a cell-seeded collagen matrix with an omental wrap. The protocol was revised once more, and the remaining 3 patients underwent implantation with cell-seeded composite collagen-PGA bladders wrapped in omentum.

The patients underwent evaluation of their genitourinary tract before proceeding with a cystogram, urodynamic study, genitourinary ultrasonography, and basic laboratory studies, including urine culture. Approximately 7 to 8 weeks before planned implantation, the patients also underwent cystoscopic evaluation and a bladder biopsy through a suprapubic incision; 1 to 2 cm^2 of bladder tissue was harvested. Muscle cells were supplemented with 10% fetal bovine serum, whereas urothelial cells were grown with keratinocyte growth medium. All cells were inspected for infectious agents until implantation. The scaffolds used ranged in size from 70 cm^2 to 150 cm^2 and were shaped like a bladder with polyglycolic sutures. A specific template was used to develop the 3D scaffold for the last 3 patients with the help of 3D computed tomographic imaging. The scaffolds were 2 mm in thickness. The exterior of the scaffolds was seeded with smooth muscle cells. The inside of the scaffolds was coated with urothelial cells 48 hours later.

The constructs were implanted in the patients 7 weeks after biopsy and after the patients had been on 7 days of oral antibiotics. A midline vertical incision was made, and the bladder was opened with a cruciate incision. A suprapubic catheter was placed, which exited via the native bladder tissue and a transurethral catheter was also left in place. The engineered bladder was sutured to native bladder tissue with 4-0 polyglycolic suture in a running fashion. One of the 4 patients who had collagen scaffolds implanted received an omental wrap of their construct, whereas all 3 patients receiving the composite scaffolds had their implants wrapped in omentum. Because the gastrointestinal tract was not violated as in enteric augmentation cystoplasties, patients did not need nasogastric suctioning, and they were started on a diet within 24 hours of surgery. The drain left in the pelvis was removed 3 to 5 days after surgery, and the first of the urinary drainage catheters was removed after performing a cystogram 3 weeks after surgery. Bladder cycling was then performed by intermittently clamping the remaining catheter for the next 14 days, after which the catheter was removed and clean intermittent catheterization was restarted. All patients were restarted on anticholinergics postoperatively.

Serial urodynamics, cystograms, ultrasonographies, and bladder biopsies were performed and serum values taken. Leak point pressure decreased in all patients; however, it decreased the most in the patients with composite-engineered bladders with an omental wrap. The mean leak point pressure at capacity decreased by 12% in the collagen-engineered bladders without an omental wrap, by 29% in the collaged-engineered bladder with an omental wrap, and by 56% in the composite-engineered bladders with an omental wrap. In fact, the patients who had the collagen composite constructs implanted with an omental wrap had lower mean bladder leak point pressures, greater capacity, greater compliance, and longer dry periods. The bladder biopsies revealed adequate structural architecture and phenotype. On cystoscopic evaluation, the margin between composite matrix-based engineered segments and the native bladders were grossly indistinguishable (**Fig. 1**).[19] This clinical trial engineered human bladder tissues for young patients with end-stage bladder disease by isolating autologous bladder urothelial and muscle cells, expanding these cells in vitro, attaching them to various biodegradable 3D matrices, and implanting the resulting tissue into

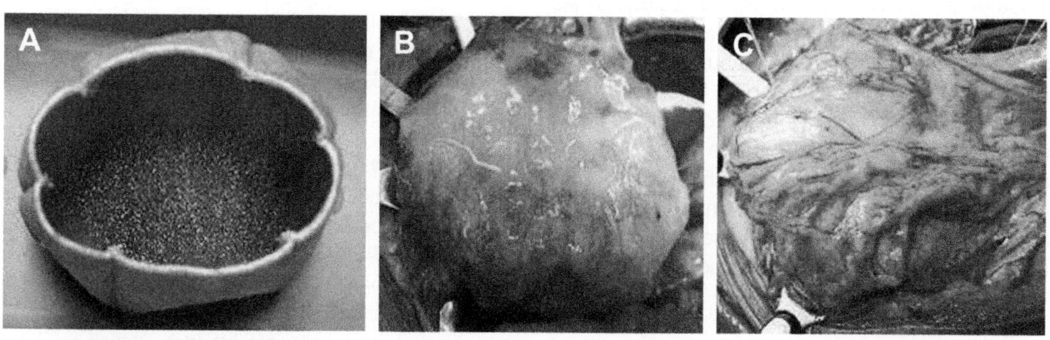

Fig. 1. Construction of engineered bladder. (*A*) Scaffold material seeded with cells for use in bladder repair. (*B*) The seeded scaffold is anastomosed to native bladder with running 4-0 poly-glycolic sutures. (*C*) Implant covered with fibrin glue and omentum. (*Courtesy of* Dr Anthony Atala, Wake Forest University Baptist Medical Center, Winston-Salem, North Carolina).

patients with or without omental wrapping. The use of composite scaffold made of PGA proved to support cell growth and survival better than collagen scaffolds and to be optimal for the engineering of bladder tissue in this trial. Also, omental wrapping proved to be beneficial. Omentum, commonly used in reconstructive surgery because of its ability to enhance neovascularization, proved to contribute to the ultimate success of the engineered bladders in this trial. The authors' clinical trial is overall the most complete clinical trial for tissue engineering to date and demonstrates the potential applications of tissue engineering to urology. This clinical experience is promising in that it showed that engineered tissues can be safely and effectively implanted in patients; however, further studies must be conducted if engineered bladders are to become the first-line option for bladder reconstruction.

SUMMARY

Much has been learned about replacement of tissue and attempts to complete an organ. Several challenges need to be addressed and refined. How to harness our unique regenerative processes and limit our evolutionary reparative powers are still being studied. Neuronal innervation and whether one can receive and transmit factors to the intact nerve system require further study. Neural constituents within the bladder tissue can be clearly identified, and transmitting information to the nervous system could improve the regenerative process. Further work also needs to be completed to determine when to incorporate growth factors into the process to maximize their contribution to the regenerative process.

Another major limitation within tissue engineering of any large construct is the ability to provide a sufficient, robust blood supply to the organ after it is implanted. Organs that are large cannot depend solely on diffusion for the delivery of nutrients and removal of waste products. As more intricate and developed organs are created and implanted, a better way to supply them with blood also needs to be developed. Should bladder tissue be prevascularized in vitro to improve function in vivo? Is there a role for gene therapy, nanoparticles, or other materials to enhance structure and function of the constructs? Continued exploration and discovery within tissue regeneration would provide answers to these questions and many more.

REFERENCES

1. Yoshimura N, Chancellor MB. Physiology and pharmacology of the bladder and urethra. In: Wein AJ, Kavoussi LR, Novick AC, et al, editors. Campbell-Walsh urology. 9th edition. Philadelphia: W.B. Sanders Company; 2007. p. 1922–72.
2. Dahl DM, McDougal WS. Use of intestinal segments in urinary diversion. In: Wein AJ, Kavoussi LR, Novick AC, et al, editors. Campbell-Walsh urology. 9th edition. Philadelphia: W.B. Sanders Company; 2007. p. 2534–78.
3. Langer R, Vacanti JP. Tissue engineering. Science 1993;260(5110):920–6.
4. Jayo MJ, Jain D, Wagner BJ, et al. Early cellular and stromal responses in regeneration versus repair of a mammalian bladder using autologous cell and biodegradable scaffold technologies. J Urol 2008; 180:392–7.
5. Hsueh-kung L, Cowan R, Moore P, et al. Characterization of neuropathic bladder smooth muscle cells in culture. J Urol 2004;171:1348–52.
6. Yu RN, Estrada CR. Stem cells: a review and implications for urology. J Urol 2010;75:664–70.
7. Evans M, Kaugman M. Establishment in culture of pluripotent cells from mouse embryos. Nature 1981;292(5819):154–6.
8. Thomson JA, Itskovitz-Eldor J, Shapiro SS, et al. Embryonic stem cell lines derived from human blastocysts. Science 1998;282:1145–7.
9. Takahashi K, Yamanaka S. Induction of pluripotent stem cells from mouse embryonic and adult fibroblast cultures by defined factors. Cell 2006;126: 663–76.
10. Yu J, Vodyanik MA, Smuga-Otto K, et al. Induced pluripotent stem cell lines derived from human somatic cells. Science 2007;318:1917–20.
11. Takahashi K, Tanabe K, Ohnuki M, et al. Induction of pluripotent stem cells from adult human fibroblasts by defined factors. Cell 2007;131:861–72.
12. De Coppi P, Bartsch G Jr, Siddiqui MM, et al. Isolation of amniotic stem cell lines with potential for therapy. Nat Biotechnol 2007;25:100–6.
13. Zhang Y, McNeill E, Tian H, et al. Urine derived cells are a potential source for urological tissue reconstruction. J Urol 2008;180:2226–33.
14. Tian H, Bharadwaj S, Liu Y, et al. Myogenic differentiation of human bone marrow mesenchymal stem cells on a 3D nano fibrous scaffold for bladder tissue engineering. Biomaterials 2010;31: 870–7.
15. Tian H, Bharadwaj S, Liu Y, et al. Differentiation of human bone marrow mesenchymal stem cells into bladder cells: potential for urological tissue engineering. Tissue Eng Part A 2010;16:1769–79.
16. Anumanthan G, Makari JH, Nonea L, et al. Directed differentiation of bone marrow derived mesenchymal stem cells into bladder urothelium. J Urol 2008;180:1778–83.
17. Zhang Y, Frimberger D, Cheng EY, et al. Challenges in a larger bladder replacement with cell-seeded

and unseeded small intestinal submucosa grafts in a subtotal cystectomy model. BJU Int 2006;98: 1100.

18. Engelhardt EM, Stegberg E, Brown RA, et al. Compressed collagen gel: a novel scaffold for human bladder cells. J Tissue Eng Regen Med 2010;4:123–30.
19. Atala A, Bauer SB, Soker S, et al. Tissue-engineered autologous bladders for patients needing cystoplasty. Lancet 2006;367:1241–6.

Urologic Complications of the Neurogenic Bladder

E. Ann Gormley, MD

KEYWORDS

- Neurogenic bladder • Urologic complications
- Hydroureteronephrosis • Urinary tract infections
- Destruction of the urethra

The goals of management in the patient with a neurogenic bladder should consist of preservation or improvement in upper tract function, absence or control of infection, and maintenance of a low-pressure bladder that is both continent and capable of emptying well. These goals are ideally achieved without an indwelling catheter or a stoma, and in a manner that is socially and vocationally acceptable to the patient. When these goals are not met, the complications that occur do so in a cascade whereby one complication leads to another complication and then to another. This article provides an overview of the urologic complications of the adult neurogenic bladder including hydronephrosis, renal failure, urinary tract infections (UTIs), calculus disease, bladder cancer, sexual dysfunction including infertility, and the destroyed bladder and urethra.

HYDRONEPHROSIS

Hydroureteronephrosis in the neurogenic patient may lead to renal deterioration, renal failure, and death. A high-pressure, poorly compliant bladder causes upper tract dilatation with or without vesicoureteral reflux.[1] McGuire and colleagues[2] first demonstrated the effect of elevated bladder pressure in patients with spina bifida when he noted that in patients with elevated bladder leak point pressures (>40 cm H_2O) there was a 68% incidence of vesicoureteral reflux and an 81% incidence of hydronephrosis. In patients with spinal cord injury Hackler and colleagues[1] compared patients with poor bladder compliance with patients with normal bladder compliance, and showed that the group with poor compliance had more vesicoureteral reflux, 39% compared with 6%, and more hydronephrosis, 64% compared with 21%. When reflux is found in patients with neurogenic disease, it contributes further to the development of hydronephrosis. Hydronephrosis may also be caused by detrusor sphincter dysynergia and calculus disease.

VESICOURETERAL REFLUX

In the adult with a neurogenic bladder the finding of vesicoureteral reflux should be looked on as a failure to control bladder pressure, therefore treatment should be aimed at lowering bladder pressure. Vesicoureteral reflux is primarily seen in spinal cord injured patients, particularly in patients with suprasacral injuries, and is seen in 17% to 25% of patients.[3] Reflux may occur with all forms of bladder management, particularly with the use of an indwelling catheter.[4] When vesicoureteral reflux is found, intermittent catheterization is the best method of bladder drainage in combination with anticholinergic drugs to lower the bladder pressure and to preserve the upper tracts.[5–7] If bladder pressure can be lowered and maintained, it is rare that vesicoureteral reflux persists. When a bladder augmentation is required to lower detrusor pressure in a patient with reflux, some surgeons perform an antirefluxing surgery at the same time. The use of surgery is somewhat debatable because if a bladder augmentation is successful and results in lower detrusor pressure,

Section of Urology, Department of Surgery, Dartmouth-Hitchcock Medical Center, 1 Medical Center Drive, Lebanon, NH 03756, USA
E-mail address: ann.gormley@hitchcock.org

Urol Clin N Am 37 (2010) 601–607
doi:10.1016/j.ucl.2010.07.002

reflux may resolve. The decision to reimplant should take into account grade of reflux because approximately 85% of Grade III or less reflux resolves, whereas approximately 66% of patients with Grade V reflux improve.[8–11] Although an antireflux procedure in a very thickened bladder may not be an easy procedure, Hayashi and colleagues[12] have reported minimal morbidity and good long-term outcomes with preservation of satisfactory renal outcome at a mean follow-up of 12 years in children with high-grade reflux.[12] Persistent reflux, especially of infected urine, increases the risk of upper tract infection, may predispose to calculi formation, and lead to renal deterioration and even death from renal disease in patients with spinal cord injury. In 1965, Hackler and colleagues[13] showed that 60% of patients with spinal cord injury who were dying of renal disease had persistent reflux. Today, with improved bladder pressure management, vesicoureteral reflux should be less of an issue.

RENAL FAILURE

Renal failure in neurogenic patients occurs because of chronic pyelonephritis, hydronephrosis, and renal stone formation.[13] Vesicoureteral reflux also contributes to renal deterioration, but a high-pressure bladder also impairs renal and ureteral emptying so that reflux does not have to be present in order for a patient with a neurogenic bladder to develop hydronephrosis. Renal deterioration is most commonly seen in spinal cord–injured patients with complete neurogenic lesions, cervical lesions with quadriplegia, and in those managed with indwelling catheters.[14–17] Patients with spina bifida are also at risk for renal deterioration, especially if they have detrusor overactivity with detrusor sphincter dysynergia, or if they have had aggressive treatment to increase their urethral resistance without management of their bladder pressure. Renal failure remains the leading cause of death in patients with spina bifida at all ages.[18]

Indwelling catheters have been associated with urinary tract infection, upper tract deterioration, and renal failure.[4,15,19,20]

Although a urinary diversion should lead to the creation of a low-pressure system, renal failure can still occur either because the diversion was performed too late after significant renal damage had occurred or because of obstruction, chronic infection, or chronic vesicoureteral reflux. Obstruction may result from ureteroileal anastomotic strictures, stomal stenosis, or poor conduit emptying. Most data on long-term complications of ileal conduits in neurogenic patients are obtained from the pediatric literature and are now considered historical because nowadays diversions are rarely performed in this patient population. These early series report that the rate of ureteroileal anastomotic stricture is 16.5% to 50% after 10 years.[21–26] It is hoped that renal deterioration and death from renal failure in the neurogenic population is becoming less frequent as urologic care continues to improve.

INFECTION

All patients with a neurogenic bladder are at risk of development of a UTI, regardless of how they manage their bladder. Poor bladder emptying is a known risk factor for development of UTI. The postvoid residual volume at which an alternative form of bladder emptying should be initiated is unknown. Dromerick and Edwards[27] have shown in a series of patients who have had a stroke that a postvoid residual of 150 mL is an independent risk factor for the development of UTI. In male patients who empty by increasing intravesical pressure, either by a Valsalva maneuver or by a Crede maneuver, reflux of urine into the prostate and seminal vesicles occurs in more than 50% of patients and can lead to other complications such as epididymo-orchitis.[28] Elderly male patients who use condom catheter drainage have been found to have a higher rate of UTI, 63%, than nonusers, 14%.[29]

The rate of bacteriuria following the introduction of a catheter is 5% to 8% for each day of catheterization, with a 100% incidence of bacteriuria with long-term indwelling catheters within 4 weeks.[30–32] Symptomatic infection is far less common than asymptomatic catheter-associated bacteriuria, but asymptomatic bacteriuria may lead to a symptomatic infection or be indiscriminately treated, which may lead to multiply resistant bacteria. Seminal vesiculitis, prostatitis, epididymitis, and orchitis may all be seen in patients with long-term urethral catheterization with blockage of the ejaculatory and prostatic ducts. Suprapubic catheterization and intermittent catheterization reduce the risk of these infections but do not completely eliminate them. The technique of intermittent catheterization, sterile intermittent catheterization, or clean intermittent catheterization (CIC) was examined in a recent Cochrane analysis, from which there does not seem to be a difference in the incidence of UTIs. The investigators also examined coated or uncoated catheters, single or multiple-use catheters, self-catheterization, or catheterization by others. Based on these data it is not possible to state that one catheter type, technique, or strategy is better than another. The studies used in this analysis had design flaws, and further well-designed studies were strongly recommended.[33]

The rate of bladder infection has been shown to decrease with increased frequency of catheterization, provided low-pressure storage is maintained. Treatment of symptomatic UTIs in the neurogenic patient involves treating with appropriate antibiotics, changing of all catheters once treatment is initiated, and ensuring that frequent complete emptying is achieved. In the patient with relapsing or persistent infections, a search for the source of infections must be undertaken and this may include a cystoscopy to rule out a stone, upper tract imaging to rule out stasis or a stone, and ensuring that the patient has changed all of their reusable catheters and is not reinfecting themselves.

CALCULUS DISEASE

Patients with neurogenic bladders are at increased risk for urinary tract calculi caused by urinary stasis, indwelling catheters, reflux, infection, and immobility. Stasis occurs in the poorly draining upper tract, generally as a result of high intravesical pressures with or without hydroureteronephrosis and reflux. The incidence of upper tract calculi is 10% to 20% in patients with spinal cord injury, and the risk continues over time, necessitating ongoing follow-up.[34,35] Treatment of upper tract calculi can be difficult owing to the poor drainage of the upper tract. Although shock wave lithotripsy may be effective at breaking a stone, the patient may be unable to clear the pieces. Ureteroscopy or a percutaneous nephrostolithotomy may represent a better treatment modality to ensure complete stone-free status postoperatively. In neurogenic patients undergoing percutaneous nephrostolithotomy the retreatment and complications rates are higher, primarily because of colonization or infections of the upper tracts. Care must be taken to ensure appropriate cultures are obtained pre- and perioperatively.[36,37]

Stasis in the bladder is seen in patients with infrequent or incomplete bladder emptying. Stasis can be seen in the patient with an indwelling catheter that does not drain well or in the patient who catheterizes infrequently or fails to empty fully. As noted, bacteriuria is common in patients with neurogenic bladders and this serves as an additional lithogenic factor. DeVivo and colleagues[38] found during an 8-year period that 36% of spinal cord–injured patients at their institution developed bladder calculi. Risk factors for stone formation in the first year included complete neurologic lesions and *Klebsiella* infections on admission. A follow-up study from the same institution showed that the incidence of bladder stones decreased to 8% from the 1970s to the 1990s. Bladder management played a role in the risk of stone formation. Patients with indwelling catheters had a 9-fold increased risk, and patients managed with CIC or a condom catheter had a 4-fold increased risk compared with continent patients who were catheter free.[39] Bladder management was also noted to play a role in the bladder stone risk by Ord and colleagues,[40] who calculated the risk of stone formation as 0% to 0.5% per year for condom catheterization with sphincterotomy, 0.2% for CIC, and 4% for patients with an indwelling catheter that increased to an annual risk of 16% following the development of 1 stone. Recurrent or persistent infection and/or persistent stone fragments likely play a role in recurrent stones. Although there are some series that conclude that the method of bladder management, particularly an indwelling catheter, does not contribute to the risk of stone formation, one needs to consider what the overall rate is in these series and when the bladder stones develop. One series that examined patients with spinal cord injury managed with suprapubic tubes found that 22% of patients developed bladder stones.[34] Another contemporary series showed an overall rate of bladder calculi in spinal cord–injured patients of 14%, with the greatest risk being in the first 6 months following injury, in contrast to other series in which the risk was noted to be ongoing years after the injury.[35,39]

A recent review of 56 studies examined variation between morbidity profiles of suprapubic catheters and CIC in older and more recent studies. It was noted in the review that if all patients are managed with anticholinergic medications, frequent catheter changes, and volume maintenance procedures, the morbidity is similar for suprapubic catheters and CIC.[41]

Bladder diverticuli may predispose some patients with neurogenic bladders to not fully empty with self-catheterization and thus form stones in the diverticuli. Foreign objects including catheters or pubic hair in the bladder also serve as a nidus for calculi formation.

Treatment of bladder calculi in the patient with a neurogenic bladder must take into account the patient's ability to fully empty. Although most bladder stones can be treated endoscopically through the urethra or via a percutaneous approach, the goal of the urologist should be to completely remove all stone particles. The bedridden patient with multiple sclerosis or the patient with a large redundant augmentation may not have complete bladder emptying, despite timely catheterization, because debris and mucus may layer out posteriorly and not be accessed with the catheter. Adequate fluid intake, careful and timely catheterization, daily irrigation, and eradication of urea-splitting organisms should be considered following the treatment of bladder calculi in the patient with a neurogenic bladder.[42]

BLADDER CANCER

The risk of bladder cancer is 16 to 28 times higher in patients with spinal cord injury than in the general population.[43] Factors that contribute to this higher risk include indwelling catheters, chronic infection, and bladder stones; however, in the series by Kalisvaart and colleagues[43] 52% of patients diagnosed with bladder cancer did not have an indwelling catheter. The most common tumors found were squamous cell carcinoma 46.9%, transitional cell carcinoma 31.3%, adenocarcinoma 9.4%, and mixed transitional and squamous cell carcinoma 12.5%, which is in keeping with historical series. In other contemporary series transitional cell carcinoma was the most common type of tumor found.[44,45] In many of these studies other risk factors, particularly cigarette smoking, were not well controlled, which may be very important given that some of these studies were performed in VA hospitals where the rate of cigarette smoking generally exceeds that of the non-VA population.

Stonehill and colleagues[46] have recommended a yearly urine microscopy and urine cytology to screen spinal cord–injured patients who have had an indwelling catheter for more than 5 years. Although urine cytology may be a useful test in the patient with additional risk factors for transitional cell carcinoma, one must remember that cytology is generally normal in patients with low-grade transitional cell carcinoma and in those with other types of bladder cancer. The sensitivity and specificity of urinary cytology for detecting bladder recurrence in patients with a history of nontransitional cell cancer has been shown to be 20% and 94.8%, making cytology a poor screening test.[47]

Routine yearly cystoscopy and biopsy in all spinal cord–injured patients 5 years following insertion of a suprapubic tube has been found to be a poor screening test, with chronic cystitis and squamous metaplasia being the most common finding.[48] In the spinal cord of an injured patient suspected of having a bladder tumor, cystoscopy alone does not suffice and biopsy is necessary to make the diagnosis, because chronic inflammatory changes or squamous metaplasia may be difficult to distinguish from cancerous changes. The patient with a spinal cord injury and a bladder cancer often presents with persistent gross hematuria, which should lead to a workup including cystoscopy and biopsy.[45] Although screening with cytology or yearly cystoscopy and biopsy has not been found to be beneficial, patients with signs or symptoms of a bladder cancer should be worked up because spinal cord–injured patients are more likely to present with muscle invasive bladder cancer, and earlier diagnosis may change the prognosis.[48]

Patients with spina bifida, regardless of the presence of a bladder augmentation, may develop bladder cancer at a young age and often present with atypical symptoms. The tumor histology is variable. Patients are often diagnosed with advanced disease leading to poor long-term survival.[49] Husmann and Rathbun[50] found a malignancy rate of 4.5% in their extensive database of augmented patients followed over 10 to 53 years. Most patients who developed a malignancy had coexisting risk factors, including a smoking history of greater than 50 pack-years or chronic immunosuppression.

SEXUAL DYSFUNCTION/INFERTILITY

Many medical conditions including diabetes, Parkinson disease, multiple sclerosis, and spinal cord injuries that are associated with the development of a neurogenic bladder can cause and contribute to the patient's sexual difficulties. Although neurologic deficits can affect all aspects of sexual function, determining the exact deficit is complicated and rarely changes management. In managing the patient with a neurogenic bladder the urologist must take into account the patient's interest in and ability to partake in sexual activity. Obviously the patient who can manage the bladder with CIC has greater freedom for expression of sexuality compared with the patient managed with an indwelling urethral catheter. The greater freedom that a patient may have when managed with a suprapubic tube or a stoma compared with a urethral catheter has to be countered by the possibility of perceptions of an altered body image.

The major sexual complication that is seen in patients with neurogenic bladder from spinal cord injury is infertility in men. Men with spinal cord injury are generally infertile because of ejaculatory dysfunction, impaired spermatogenesis, and poor semen quality.[51,52] Poor semen quality consisting primarily of abnormal sperm motility and viability is seen as early as 2 weeks after injury.[52] In the series by Ohl and colleagues[53] of spinal cord–injured patients undergoing electroejaculation, sperm quality was abnormal in all patients. Patients managed with intermittent catheterization had slightly better sperm quality.

Urinary infection was associated with slightly lower sperm quality and lower pregnancy rates.

THE DESTROYED BLADDER AND/OR URETHRA

CIC, although the recommended modality for bladder emptying, is not without its own complications. Urethral lesions are rare in girls and women.[54] In boys and men complications in patients on CIC for a minimum of 10 years are rare, but may include urethral lesions including the development of false passages, stricture disease, and epididymitis.[55] Stricture formation with a longer follow-up has been noted by other investigators.[39] All patients who perform CIC, whether they have been catheterizing since childhood or they are just starting, need to be provided with appropriate supplies and instructions on catheterizing, cleaning of catheters, signs of complications, and information on where and when to call to ask questions or report problems.

Long-term use of an indwelling urethral catheter may lead to urethral strictures, periurethral abscesses, urethral diverticuli, urethrocutaneous fistula formation, and erosion. Urethral strictures are common and usually extensive. Before repair of any of these complications the patient's urinary tract must be evaluated and a discussion should occur with the patient as to how their neurogenic bladder should ideally be managed both to prevent a recurrence of the problem and to prevent other problems.

A devastating complication is traumatic hypospadias, which may be limited to the glans (**Fig. 1**) or can extend to involve the urethra (**Fig. 2**). The female urethra is also at risk for erosion from a chronic indwelling catheter. Unfortunately, when these patients with urethral erosion are switched from an indwelling urethral catheter to a suprapubic tube, many continue to leak urine from the urethra if they have a high-pressure bladder and/or a patulous, eroded bladder neck. Surgical reconstruction is a formidable challenge and generally requires multiple procedures, particularly in the female patient.[56] Recurrent erosions can occur as early as 1 month postoperatively and are attributed to catheter traction.[57] In the patient with a urethral and bladder neck erosion and a small-capacity, high-pressure bladder that is debilitated with comorbidities such as osteomyelitis or severe decubiti, a urinary diversion may be necessary to achieve continence quickly.

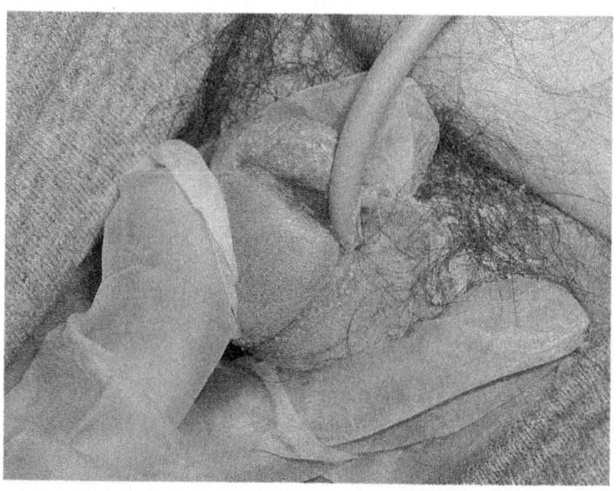

Fig. 1. A 45-year-old patient with quadriplegia shows glandular erosion after 6 months with an indwelling catheter. Note the diaper dermatitis on the glans from chronic incontinence.

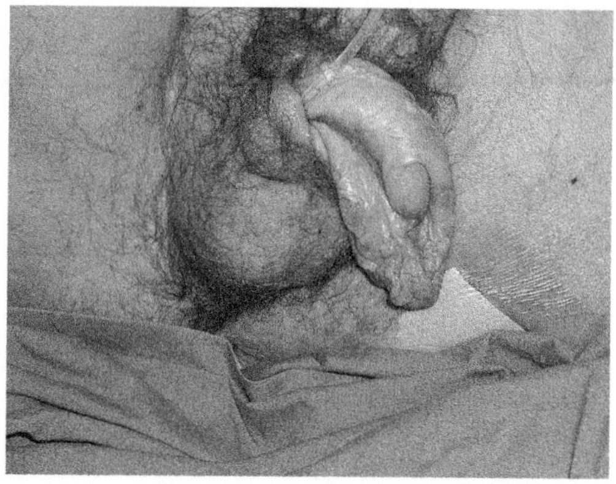

Fig. 2. A 24-year-old patient with spina bifida shows complete erosion of the urethra following 2 years with an indwelling catheter. The erosion involved the urethra and extended to the bladder neck.

SUMMARY

Patients with a neurogenic bladder are at risk for several urologic complications because of both their disease and the method by which they manage their bladder. Complications include but are not limited to hydronephrosis, renal failure, UTIs, calculus disease, bladder cancer, sexual dysfunction including infertility, and the destroyed bladder and urethra. Management of filling bladder pressures and regular, complete emptying, ideally with CIC, can prevent or delay many of these complications. Despite good urologic management, patients can develop complications over time, necessitating regular urologic follow-up with the goal of preventing further complications and ultimately preserving renal function while maintaining continence.

REFERENCES

1. Hackler RH, Hall MK, Zampieri TA. Bladder hypocompliance in the spinal cord injury population. J Urol 1989;141(6):1390–3.
2. McGuire EJ, Woodside JR, Borden TA, et al. Prognostic value of urodynamic testing in myelodysplastic patients. J Urol 1981;126(2):205–9.
3. Thomas DG, Lucas MG. The urinary tract following spinal cord injury. In: Chisolm GD, Fair WR, editors. Scientific foundations of urology. Chicago: Year Book Medical; 1990. p. 286–99.
4. Lamid S. Long-term follow-up of spinal cord injury patients with vesicoureteral reflux. Paraplegia 1988;26(1):27–34.
5. Diokno AC, Sonda LP, Hollander JB, et al. Fate of patients started on clean intermittent self-catheterization therapy 10 years ago. J Urol 1983; 129(6):1120–2.
6. McGuire EJ, Savastano JA. Long-term followup of spinal cord injury patients managed by intermittent catheterization. J Urol 1983;129(4):775–6.
7. Wyndaele JJ, Maes D. Clean intermittent self-catheterization: a 12-year followup. J Urol 1990; 143(5):906–8.
8. Simforoosh N, Tabibi A, Basiri A, et al. Is ureteral reimplantation necessary during augmentation cystoplasty in patients with neurogenic bladder and vesicoureteral reflux? J Urol 2002;168:1439–41.
9. Lopez Pereira P, Martinez Urrutia MJ, Lobato Romera R, et al. Should we treat vesicoureteral reflux in patients who simultaneously undergo bladder augmentation for neuropathic bladder? J Urol 2001; 165:2259–61.
10. Soylet Y, Emir H, Ilce Z, et al. Quo vadis? Ureteric reimplantation or ignoring reflux during augmentation cystoplasty. BJU Int 2004;94:379–80.
11. Nasrallah PF, Aliabadi HA. Bladder augmentation in patients with neurogenic bladder and vesicoureteral reflux. J Urol 1991;146:563–6.
12. Hayashi Y, Kato Y, Okazaki T, et al. The effectiveness of ureteric reimplantation during bladder augmentation for high-grade vesicoureteric reflux in patients with neurogenic bladder: long-term outcome. J Pediatr Surg 2007;42:1998–2001.
13. Hackler RH, Dalton JJ Jr, Bunts RC. Changing concepts in the preservation of renal function in the paraplegic. J Urol 1965;94:107–11.
14. Donnelly J, Hackler RH, Bunts RC. Present urologic status of the World War II paraplegic: 25-year followup. Comparison with status of the 20-year Korean War paraplegic and 5-year Vietnam paraplegic. J Urol 1972;108(4):558–62.
15. Geisler WO, Jousse AT, Wynne-Jones M, et al. Survival in traumatic spinal cord injury. Paraplegia 1983;21(6):364–73.
16. Hackler RH. A 25-year prospective mortality study in the spinal cord injured patient: comparison with the long-term living paraplegic. J Urol 1977;117(4):486–8.
17. Webb DR, Fitzpatrick JM, O'Flynn JD. A 15-year follow-up of 406 consecutive spinal cord injuries. Br J Urol 1984;56(6):614–7.
18. Woodhouse CR. Myelomeningocele in young adults. BJU Int 2005;95(2):223–30.
19. Hutch JA. Vesico-ureteral reflux in the paraplegic: cause and correction. J Urol 1952;68(2):457–69.
20. Stover SL, Lloyd LK, Waites KB, et al. Urinary tract infection in spinal cord injury. Arch Phys Med Rehabil 1989;70(1):47–54.
21. Malek RS, Burke EC, Deweerd JH. Ileal conduit urinary diversion in children. J Urol 1971;105: 892–900.
22. Schwarz GR, Jeffs RD. Ileal conduit urinary diversion in children: computer analysis of followup from 2 to 16 years. J Urol 1975;114:285–8.
23. Heath AL, Eckstein HB. Ileal conduit urinary diversion in children. A long term follow up. J Urol (Paris) 1984;90:91–6.
24. Pitts WR Jr, Muecke EC. A 20-year experience with ileal conduits: the fate of the kidneys. J Urol 1979; 122:154–7.
25. Shapiro SR, Lebowitz R, Colodny AH. Fate of 90 children with ileal conduit urinary diversion a decade later: analysis of complications, pyelography, renal function and bacteriology. J Urol 1975;114:289–95.
26. Arnarson O, Straffon RA. Clinical experience with the ileal conduit in children. J Urol 1969;102: 768–71.
27. Dromerick AW, Edwards DF. Relation of postvoid residual to urinary tract infection during stroke rehabilitation. Arch Phys Med Rehabil 2003;84(9): 1369–72.
28. Wynedaele JJ, Castro D, Madersbacher H, et al. Neurogenic and faecal incontinence. In: Abrams P, Cardozo L, Khoury S, et al, editors. Incontinence. 2nd edition. Paris: Health Publications Ltd; 2005. p. 1059–362.
29. Johnson JR, Roberts PL, Olsen RJ, et al. Prevention of catheter associated urinary tract infection with a silver oxide-coated urinary catheter: clinical and microbiologic correlates. J Infect Dis 1990;162(5): 1145–50.
30. Mulhall AB, Chapman RG, Crow RA. Bacteruria during indwelling urethral catheterization. J Hosp Infect 1988;11(3):253–62.
31. Stamm WE. Catheter-associated urinary tract infections: epidemiology, pathogenesis, and prevention. Am J Med 1991;91(3B):65S–71S.
32. Nicolle LE. The chronic indwelling catheter and urinary infection in long-term-care facility residents. Infect Control Hosp Epidemiol 2001;22(5): 316–21.

33. Moore KN, Fader M, Getliffe K. Long-term bladder management by intermittent catheterization in adults and children. Cochrane Database Syst Rev 2007;4: CD006008.
34. Sugimura T, Arnold E, English S, et al. Chronic suprapubic catheterization in the management of patients with spinal cord injuries: analysis of upper and lower urinary tract complications. BJU Int 2008;101(11):1396–400.
35. Hansen RB, Biering-Sorensen F, Kristensen JK. Urinary calculi following traumatic spinal cord injury. Scand J Urol Nephrol 2007;41(2):115–9.
36. Ost MC, Lee BR. Urolithiasis in patients with spinal cord injuries: risk factors, management, and outcomes. Curr Opin Urol 2006;16(2):93–9.
37. Rubenstein JN, Gonzalez CM, Blunt LW, et al. Safety and efficacy of percutaneous nephrolithotomy in patients with neurogenic bladder dysfunction. Urology 2004;63(4):636–40.
38. DeVivo MJ, Fine PR, Cutter GR, et al. The risk of bladder calculi in patients with spinal cord injuries. Arch Intern Med 1985;145(3):428–30.
39. Chen Y, DeVivo MJ, Lloyd LK. Bladder stone incidence in persons with spinal cord injury: determinants and trends, 1973-1996. Urology 2001;58(5): 665–70.
40. Ord J, Lunn D, Reynard J. Bladder management and risk of bladder stone formation in spinal cord injured patients. J Urol 2003;170(5):1734–7.
41. Feifer A, Corcos J. Contemporary role of suprapubic cystostomy in treatment of neuropathic bladder dysfunction in spinal cord injured patients. Neurourol Urodyn 2008;27(6):475–9.
42. Kronner KM, Casale AJ, Cain MP, et al. Bladder calculi in the pediatric augmented bladder. J Urol 1998;160(3 Pt 2):1096–8 [discussion: 1103].
43. Kalisvaart JF, Katsumi HK, Ronningen LD, et al. Bladder cancer in spinal cord injury patients. Spinal Cord 2010;48(3):257–61.
44. Hess MJ, Zhan EH, Foo DK, et al. Bladder cancer in patients with spinal cord injury. J Spinal Cord Med 2003;26(4):335–8.
45. Pannek J. Transitional cell carcinoma in patients with spinal cord injury: a high risk malignancy? Urology 2002;59(2):240–4.
46. Stonehill WH, Dmochowski RR, Patterson AL, et al. Risk factors for bladder tumors in spinal cord injury patients. J Urol 1996;155(4):1248–50.
47. Hutterer GC, Karakiewicz PI, Zippe C, et al. Urinary cytology and nuclear matrix protein 22 in the detection of bladder cancer recurrence other than transitional cell carcinoma. BJU Int 2008;101(5):561–5.
48. Hamid R, Bycroft J, Arya M, et al. Screening cystoscopy and biopsy in patients with neuropathic bladder and chronic suprapubic indwelling catheters: is it valid? J Urol 2003;170(2 Pt 1):425–7.
49. Austin JC, Elliott S, Cooper CS. Patients with spina bifida and bladder cancer: atypical presentation, advanced stage and poor survival. J Urol 2007; 178(3 Pt 1):798–801.
50. Husmann DA, Rathbun SR. Long-term follow up of enteric bladder augmentations: the risk for malignancy. J Pediatr Urol 2008;4(5):381–5 [discussion: 386].
51. Monga M, Bernie J, Rajasekaran M. Male infertility and erectile dysfunction in spinal cord injury: a review. Arch Phys Med Rehabil 1999;80(10): 1331–9.
52. Patki P, Woodhouse J, Hamid R, et al. Effects of spinal cord injury on semen parameters. J Spinal Cord Med 2008;31(1):27–32.
53. Ohl DA, Denil J, Fitzgerald-Shelton K, et al. Fertility of spinal cord injured males: effect of genitourinary infection and bladder management on results of electroejaculation. J Am Paraplegia Soc 1992;15(2):53–9.
54. Lindehall B, Abrahamsson K, Jodal U, et al. Complications of clean intermittent catheterization in young females with myelomeningocele: 10 to 19 years of followup. J Urol 2007;178:1053–5.
55. Lindehall B, Abrahamsson K, Hjalmas K, et al. Complications of clean intermittent catheterization in boys and young males with neurogenic bladder dysfunction. J Urol 2004;172:1686–8.
56. Stoffel JT, McGuire EJ. Outcome of urethral closure in patients with neurologic impairment and complete urethral destruction. Neurourol Urodyn 2006;25(1): 19–22.
57. Meeks JJ, Erickson BA, Helfand BT, et al. Reconstruction of urethral erosion in men with a neurogenic bladder. BJU Int 2009;103(3):378–81.

Index

Note: Page numbers of article titles are in **boldface** type.

Urol Clin N Am 37 (2010) 609–614
doi:10.1016/S0094-0143(10)00094-7
0094-0143/10/$ – see front matter

V

X

United States Postal Service

Statement of Ownership, Management, and Circulation (All Periodicals Publications Except Requestor Publications)

1. Publication Title: Urologic Clinics of North America	2. Publication Number: 0 0 0 - 7 1 1	3. Filing Date: 9/15/10
4. Issue Frequency: Feb, May, Aug, Nov	5. Number of Issues Published Annually: 4	6. Annual Subscription Price: $291.00

7. Complete Mailing Address of Known Office of Publication (*Not printer*) (*Street, city, county, state, and ZIP+4®*)

Elsevier Inc.
360 Park Avenue South
New York, NY 10010-1710

Contact Person: Stephen Bushing
Telephone (Include area code): 215-239-3688

8. Complete Mailing Address of Headquarters or General Business Office of Publisher (*Not printer*)

Elsevier Inc., 360 Park Avenue South, New York, NY 10010-1710

9. Full Names and Complete Mailing Addresses of Publisher, Editor, and Managing Editor (*Do not leave blank*)

Publisher (*Name and complete mailing address*)

Kim Murphy, Elsevier, Inc., 1600 John F. Kennedy Blvd. Suite 1800, Philadelphia, PA 19103-2899

Editor (*Name and complete mailing address*)

Kerry Holland, Elsevier, Inc., 1600 John F. Kennedy Blvd. Suite 1800, Philadelphia, PA 19103-2899

Managing Editor (*Name and complete mailing address*)

Catherine Bewick, Elsevier, Inc., 1600 John F. Kennedy Blvd. Suite 1800, Philadelphia, PA 19103-2899

10. Owner (*Do not leave blank. If the publication is owned by a corporation, give the name and address of the corporation immediately followed by the names and addresses of all stockholders owning or holding 1 percent or more of the total amount of stock. If not owned by a corporation, give the names and addresses of the individual owners. If owned by a partnership or other unincorporated firm, give its name and address as well as those of each individual owner. If the publication is published by a nonprofit organization, give its name and address.*)

Full Name	Complete Mailing Address
Wholly owned subsidiary of	4520 East-West Highway
Reed/Elsevier, US holdings	Bethesda, MD 20814

11. Known Bondholders, Mortgagees, and Other Security Holders Owning or Holding 1 Percent or More of Total Amount of Bonds, Mortgages, or Other Securities. If none, check box → ☐ None

Full Name	Complete Mailing Address
N/A	

12. Tax Status (*For completion by nonprofit organizations authorized to mail at nonprofit rates*) (*Check one*)
The purpose, function, and nonprofit status of this organization and the exempt status for federal income tax purposes:
☐ Has Not Changed During Preceding 12 Months
☐ Has Changed During Preceding 12 Months (*Publisher must submit explanation of change with this statement*)

PS Form 3526, September 2007 (Page 1 of 3 (Instructions Page 3)) PSN 7530-01-000-9931 **PRIVACY NOTICE**: See our Privacy policy in www.usps.com

13. Publication Title: Urologic Clinics of North America

14. Issue Date for Circulation Data Below: August 2010

15. Extent and Nature of Circulation		Average No. Copies Each Issue During Preceding 12 Months	No. Copies of Single Issue Published Nearest to Filing Date
a. Total Number of Copies (*Net press run*)		2925	2800
b. Paid Circulation (By Mail and Outside the Mail)	(1) Mailed Outside-County Paid Subscriptions Stated on PS Form 3541. (*Include paid distribution above nominal rate, advertiser's proof copies, and exchange copies*)	1034	970
	(2) Mailed In-County Paid Subscriptions Stated on PS Form 3541 (*Include paid distribution above nominal rate, advertiser's proof copies, and exchange copies*)		
	(3) Paid Distribution Outside the Mails Including Sales Through Dealers and Carriers, Street Vendors, Counter Sales, and Other Paid Distribution Outside USPS®	815	834
	(4) Paid Distribution by Other Classes Mailed Through the USPS (e.g. First-Class Mail®)		
c. Total Paid Distribution (*Sum of 15b (1), (2), (3), and (4)*) ►		1849	1804
d. Free or Nominal Rate Distribution (By Mail and Outside the Mail)	(1) Free or Nominal Rate Outside-County Copies Included on PS Form 3541	130	86
	(2) Free or Nominal Rate In-County Copies Included on PS Form 3541		
	(3) Free or Nominal Rate Copies Mailed at Other Classes Through the USPS (e.g. First-Class Mail)		
	(4) Free or Nominal Rate Distribution Outside the Mail (Carriers or other means)		
e. Total Free or Nominal Rate Distribution (Sum of 15d (1), (2), (3) and (4)		130	86
f. Total Distribution (Sum of 15c and 15e) ►		1979	1890
g. Copies not Distributed (See instructions to publishers #4 (page #3)) ►		946	910
h. Total (Sum of 15f and g)		2925	2800
i. Percent Paid (15c divided by 15f times 100) ►		93.43%	95.45%

16. Publication of Statement of Ownership

If the publication is a general publication, publication of this statement is required. Will be printed in the **November 2010** issue of this publication. Publication not required

17. Signature and Title of Editor, Publisher, Business Manager, or Owner

Stephen R. Bushing – Fulfillment/Inventory Specialist

Date: September 15, 2010

I certify that all information furnished on this form is true and complete. I understand that anyone who furnishes false or misleading information on this form or who omits material or information requested on the form may be subject to criminal sanctions (including fines and imprisonment) and/or civil sanctions (including civil penalties).

PS Form 3526, September 2007 (Page 2 of 3)

Printed and bound by CPI Group (UK) Ltd, Croydon, CR0 4YY
03/10/2024
01040354-0012